SOCIAL WORK AND DIRECT PAYMENTS

Jon Glasby and Rosemary Littlechild

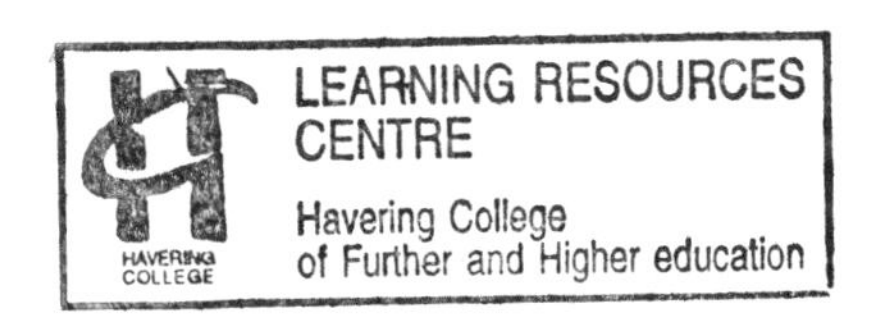

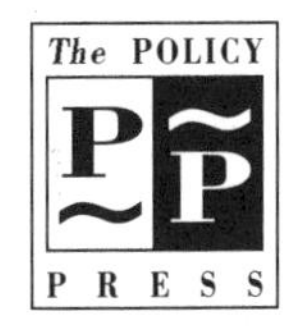

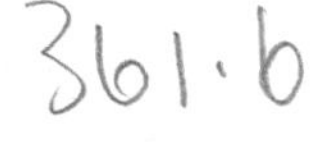

First published in Great Britain in July 2002 by

The Policy Press
34 Tyndall's Park Road
Bristol BS8 1PY
UK

Tel +44 (0)117 954 6800
Fax +44 (0)117 973 7308
e-mail tpp@bristol.ac.uk
www.policypress.org.uk

British Library Cataloguing in Publication Data
A catalogue record for this book is available from the British Library

ISBN 1 86134 385 X paperback
A hardcover version of this book is also available

Jon Glasby is a Lecturer in the Health Services Management Centre, University of Birmingham and **Rosemary Littlechild** is a Lecturer in Social Work at the Department of Social Policy and Social Work, University of Birmingham.

Cover design by Qube Design Associates, Bristol.
Front cover: photograph supplied by the Institute on Independent Living, Sweden

The Policy Press works to counter discrimination on grounds of gender, race, disability, age and sexuality.

Printed and bound in Great Britain by Bell & Bain Ltd, Glasgow.

Contents

List of tables and boxes

Tables

Boxes

Foreword

This book charts a profound change in the relationship between disabled people and the welfare state. The impact of direct payments may only be marginal as yet, but their potential is growing ever larger. They may in time reshape the entire provision of social care.

Direct payments are based on a disarmingly simple idea: that what stops disabled people from being independent is a lack of control over the services that support them. If they can control the budget being spent on their behalf, they can choose support staff that suit them individually. Such a simple idea challenges the traditional view of disabled people as vulnerable and dependent on others.

Direct payments are an example of a social policy developed by users and subsequently taken up with enthusiasm by government. But, as this book shows, turning a grassroots initiative into a national policy option involves a lot of trial and error, and we are still at a point of testing some of the practice ideas.

Setting direct payments in context, as well as explaining the current law and policy advice, is an important element in this book. Jon Glasby and Rosemary Littlechild have reviewed a wide range of material on direct payments and gathered it in one volume for the first time.

I welcome this addition to the direct payments literature, because it will help to spread this simple but revolutionary idea more widely. I hope it will help to take direct payments into the mainstream of social care. Direct payments matter because they offer the choice of independent living. It is my dream that every disabled person has this choice in future.

Frances Hasler
Director, National Centre for Independent Living

Acknowledgements

No book can be written in isolation and many people have contributed to this publication. In particular, the authors are grateful to Age Concern England, Colin Barnes, Stuart Baxter, Catherine Bewley, the British Institute of Learning Disabilities, the British Council of Disabled People, Wendy Brown, Gary Craig, Deborah Davidson, the Department of Health, the Department of Health Social Services and Public Safety, the Disablement Income Group, David Ellis, Renee Francis, Debbie Garft, the Independent Living Fund, MIND, the National AIDS Trust, the National Centre for Independent Living, the National Development Team, the North West Training and Development Team, Charlotte Pearson, the Policy Studies Institute, Cath Riley, Martin Routledge, the Scottish Executive, Simon Stockton, the UK Advocacy Network, Values Into Action, the Welsh Assembly and Guy Wishart.

Above all, the authors wish to thank Frances Hasler, Andrew Rowe and Roy Taylor.

Although a range of organisations and individuals have provided information for this book, the views expressed remain those of the authors alone.

List of abbreviations

ACAS	Advisory, Conciliation and Arbitration Service
ADSS	Association of Directors of Social Services
BCODP	British Council of Disabled People
CIL	Centre for Independent Living
CIPFA	Chartered Institute of Public Finance and Accountancy
COS	Charity Organisation Society
DoH	Department of Health
DHSSPS	Department of Health, Social Services and Public Safety
DIG	Disablement Income Group
EACHH	European Association for Care and Help at Home
ENIL	European Network on Independent Living
HSE	Health and Safety Executive
ILF	Independent Living Fund
NCIL	National Centre for Independent Living
NWTDT	North West Training and Development Team
PA	Personal Assistant
PAYE	Pay As You Earn
PSI	Policy Studies Institute
SI	Statutory Instrument
SR	Statutory Rule
SSI	Social Services Inspectorate
TAG	Technical Advisory Group
VIA	Values into Action

Note: References to parliamentary sources are given by means of the following abbreviations: HCD (House of Commons Debates), HLD (House of Lords Debates) and SC (Standing Committee, with the committee letter in brackets).

ONE

Introduction

Background and aims

The 1996 Community Care (Direct Payments) Act, which came into force on 1 April 1997, has been described as holding out "the potential for the most fundamental reorganisation of welfare for half a century" (Oliver and Sapey, 1999, p 175). After longstanding pressure from a range of user groups, the Act empowered social services departments to make cash payments to service users aged between 18 and 65 in lieu of direct service provision. Although progress has since been slow, more and more authorities have begun to implement direct payment schemes and the original Act has been extended to include older people, younger people aged 16 and 17, carers and the parents of disabled children. As recent research has begun to highlight the strengths and weaknesses of direct payments, a comprehensive introductory text is required to guide practitioners through the issues at stake in this fundamental area of practice, summarising current knowledge about good practice and exploring the implications of direct payments, both for service users and for social work staff.

Against this background, *Social work and direct payments* seeks to:

- review the history of direct payments, from the rise of the Independent Living Movement, through indirect payments to the 1996 Direct Payments Act and subsequent extensions to other user groups (Chapters Two to Four);
- chart the progress of direct payments and the pace of implementation (Chapter Five);
- explore the experience of different user groups and the relevance of issues such as ethnicity and sexuality (Chapter Six);
- examine the advantages and limitations of direct payments (Chapters Seven and Eight);
- review the practical issues which managing direct payments raises (Chapter Nine);
- identify the implications for policy makers and social workers (Chapter Ten);
- outline useful resources for those interested in finding out more about direct payments (Appendix).

Current literature

At the time of writing (2001), there has not yet been a comprehensive introductory book on the topic. Despite this, *Social work and direct payments* draws on three main types of literature:

1. *Official guidance:* policy and practice guidance produced by the Department of Health (DoH) (1997a, 2000a) provides detailed guidelines about the implementation and purpose of direct payments. This is accompanied by easily accessible guidance for users with learning difficulties (DoH, 2000b) and a number of information videos (DoH, 1998c, 1999). Further sources of official guidance are set out in the Appendix.
2. *Empirical research:* to date, a number of research studies have begun to identify the advantages and potential limitations of direct payments, highlighting the different experiences of different user groups. Thus, large-scale surveys conducted by the Association of Directors of Social Services (ADSS) (Jones, 2000) and the Scottish Executive (Witcher et al, 2000) have charted the pace of change as more and more authorities develop direct payment schemes. At the same time, more qualitative, user-focused research has started to explore the experience of service users, practitioners and personal assistants (see, for example, Holman and Bewley, 1999; Dawson, 2000; Fruin, 2000; Glendinning et al, 2000a).
3. *Practical advice/'grey' literature:* a number of organisations of disabled people produce practical information about employment legislation, health and safety and setting up support schemes. Relevant organisations include the British Council of Disabled People (BCODP), the Disablement Income Group (DIG), the National Centre for Independent Living and the West of England Centre for Integrated Living (see, for example, Dunne with Hoyle, 1992; ILSA, 1998; Vasey, 2000). While much of this material is formally published and very well publicised, some sources are Internet-based (see, for example, Morris, 1995) while others are relatively unknown and much harder to obtain.

By themselves, each of these sources provides only a limited insight into the issues which direct payments raise and there is an urgent need for an introductory publication to summarise our existing knowledge and explore the implications of direct payments for service users and frontline practitioners. It is this gap in the current literature that *Social work and direct payments* seeks to fill.

Terminology

As non-disabled writers addressing a topic of considerable interest to disabled people, terminology is crucial. Language can be a significant mechanism in constructing and maintaining oppression, both through overtly discriminatory words and through more subtle, insidious processes (Thompson, 1997). As a result, *Social work and direct payments* follows disabled writers such as Morris (1993a), or Oliver (1990, 1996) in adopting a social model of disability. Whereas previous medical approaches have tended to focus on the physical limitations of individuals, the social model of disability emphasises the physical and attitudinal barriers which exclude disabled people from participating fully in society (Oliver, 1990). Thus, the focus of intervention should be the current social organisation rather than the individual. Central to the social model is the distinction between two key concepts (Oliver, 1990, p 11):

1. *Impairment:* lacking part or all of a limb; or having a defective limb, organism or mechanism of the body.
2. *Disability:* the disadvantage or restriction of activity caused by a contemporary social organisation which takes little or no account of people who have physical impairments and thus excludes them from the mainstream of social activities.

As a result, disabled writers have tended to advocate the use of terms such as *disabled people* to refer to the oppression which people with impairments experience as a result of prejudice and discrimination:

> People are disabled by society's reaction to impairment; this is why the term disabled people is used, rather than people with disabilities. The latter term really means people with impairments whereas the disability movement prefers to use the politically more powerful term, disabled people, in order to place the emphasis on how society oppresses people with a whole range of impairments. (Morris, 1993a, p x)

In keeping with this approach, *Social work and direct payments* uses the term *disabled people* to refer to all people with an impairment, retaining *people with physical impairments* as a technical term to distinguish such service users from other user groups (such as people with learning difficulties or people with mental health problems).

TWO

History

To understand how fundamental the introduction of direct payments has been, it is necessary to have a basic awareness of the history of social work and its relationship with financial/poverty issues. As a result, this chapter begins with a brief consideration of the origins of modern social work in 19th-century philanthropy and the now notorious Poor Law, before providing a more detailed analysis of the build-up to the 1996 Community Care (Direct Payments) Act.

Social work and finance/poverty

The Charity Organisation Society

Social work, as a profession, has its origins in 19th-century philanthropy and in the pioneering approach of the Charity Organisation Society (COS) (Bosanquet, 1914; Rooff, 1972; Walton, 1975; Lewis, 1995). Founded in 1869 by a group of individuals that included Octavia Hill, the renowned housing reformer and a founder member of the National Trust, COS was essentially a reaction against a recent proliferation of philanthropic activity following the depression of the late 1860s. By offering charity to the poor, it was argued, the rich were encouraging them to become dependent on alms and exacerbating rather than resolving the problem. For leading COS figures such as Charles Loch or Helen Bosanquet, poverty was caused by individual and moral failings – by fecklessness and thriftlessness. As a result, the solution lay in individual casework, with a COS worker assessing whether an individual was worthy or unworthy of assistance. For those deemed deserving, access to charitable resources might be permitted, although the emphasis was still very much on the need for moral reformation and for the individual to change and improve their ways. For the undeserving, charity should be denied and the applicant left to rely on the harsh mechanism of the Poor Law and the workhouse. Although relatively little is known about the reaction of the poor to this form of charity, it seems likely that many felt aggrieved by this patronising and highly judgemental approach to poverty and reacted angrily to COS workers. Certainly when an East End clergyman and his wife sought to abolish almsgiving and establish a local COS, they were besieged by an angry mob on more than one occasion. In the end, such demonstrations became so widespread that the clergyman had to cut a door from the vicarage to his church so that he could slip out and fetch the police whenever the mob gathered outside (Barnett, 1918, p 84).

The Poor Law

For those deemed undeserving of COS assistance, the only other option was the Poor Law. Associated with legislation from the reign of Elizabeth I, the Poor Law levied poor rates and provided support to those in need via the workhouse and via outdoor relief. As Englander explains:

> Outdoor relief ... embraced payments for all sorts and conditions – weekly pensions to the aged and infirm, payments for the foster care of village orphans and the upkeep of illegitimate children; casual doles for those in need due to unemployment or sickness; payments for doctor's bills and grants of food, fuel and clothing, particularly during periods of dearth. (Englander, 1998, pp 2-3)

Although outdoor relief was technically abolished in 1834, it continued to be paid in practice well into the 20th century (Fraser, 1984; Novak, 1988; Rose, 1988), and was later extended during the 1920s and 1930s to include a complex range of measures to support the poor during the Great Depression (Thane, 1996). Despite this, the Poor Law is most associated with the brutal and dehumanising regime of the workhouse. To ensure that state support did not encourage the able-bodied to become idle, the Poor Law Amendment Act of 1834 introduced the concept of 'less eligibility' (that is, that the workhouse should be made as harsh as possible so that residents were less well off than even the poorest workers outside the workhouse):

> To this end, indoor relief was made as disagreeable as possible by vexatious regulations, want of social amenities, hard labour, poor dietaries and the impact of strict discipline. (Englander, 1998, pp 11-12)

Rising at 6 am in the summer and 8 am in the winter, inmates worked until 6 pm, families were separated and distinctive uniforms were enforced to emphasise 'pauper' status and advertise residents' shame (Englander, 1998). Hardly surprisingly, such institutions were bitterly resented by the working classes, many of whom would rather have starved than enter the workhouse (Chinn, 1995). As a result, the 1834 Poor Law Amendment Act was greeted with widespread rioting (Edsall, 1971) and the brutality of the Poor Law has been immortalised by writers such as Charles Dickens (1867).

As unemployment soared in the 1920s and 1930s, new sources of financial assistance were introduced to provide support for the poor (Fraser, 1984). In the 1920s, attempts were made to reduce the cost of such support through the introduction of a stringent 'means test' and the 'genuinely seeking work' test (Thane, 1996). Henceforth, all applicants for state support would have their finances and situations fully assessed, only receiving payments if they were extremely impoverished and if no other source of support was available. Once again, such intrusion into the lives of the poor was heavily resented (Thane, 1996), and the oppressive nature of the system has been widely condemned in literature such as Greenwood's *Love on the dole* (1969).

The abolition of the Poor Law

As pressure mounted to reform the Poor Law in the 1930s and early 1940s, there was a growing awareness that social work should seek to distance itself from its 19th century origins in order to rid itself of the taint of the Poor Law. Thus, when the Poor Law was finally abolished in 1948, it was replaced by a national scheme for the payment of social security benefits and by new legislation to provide welfare services for older and disabled people. For the first time in its history, social work was separated from the administration of income support and, unlike most other European countries and the US (Davis and Stephenson, 1999), social care workers were to play no active part in assessing eligibility for social security payments:

> [The National Assistance Act 1948] repealed the old Poor Law and replaced it with assistance provided by the National Assistance Board and local authorities. Whereas the Poor Law had dealt with the financial and non-financial welfare of those in need, this Act now divided these up: financial welfare was to be dealt with by the National Assistance Board, whereas it was now the responsibility of local authorities to deal with the non-financial welfare of disabled people, older people and others. Thus, the system developed a sharp separation between cash and in-kind assistance. Social security was to be about the provision of cash, subject to national rules. The social services were to operate locally and apply a much greater degree of discretion in their day-to-day work. This split is not typically found in continental Europe, where local social workers are often involved in the payment of cash benefits. (McKay and Rowlingson, 1999, p 59)

At the time, the separation of social work and social security was seen as a major advance, since social workers would be able to support those in need without the stigma of the old Poor Law (Jordan, 1974). With hindsight, however, the attempt to distance social work from cash payments to those in need has been responsible for practitioners' subsequent failure to address poverty issues. Although the vast majority of people who use social work services are in receipt of social security benefits, many social workers have tended to distance themselves from the material difficulties of their clients and have little "poverty awareness" (Becker, 1997, p 93), viewing money problems as being the responsibility of other agencies (see Box 1). This has contributed to a rapid expansion in specialist money advice services from the early 1970s onwards. From the foundation of the first Money Advice Centre in 1969 (Glasby, 1999), large numbers of services have been established throughout the UK to support people with financial problems. By 1989, there were 221 voluntary organisations providing such services, while local authorities operated a further 40 schemes, often via specialist units or advisers rather than through social services departments (Kempson, 1995, pp 3-4). Despite a growing awareness of the importance of poverty issues (see, for example, Becker and MacPherson, 1988;

Box 1: The lack of poverty awareness

Social work trainers in Birmingham working in the field of mental health ask students why most people they work with face problems associated with poverty such as debt, homelessness, inadequate diets, insufficient clothing and lack of social contacts. Common responses include:

- Poverty is "a fact of life for people like this".
- "It's not our job to tackle poverty."
- "The mentally ill bring it on themselves."
- "People like this should be grateful for what they get" and "count their blessings".
- "If these people were given more they would only waste it."

(Davis and Wainwright, 1996, p 49)

Burgess, 1994; Davis and Wainwright, 1996), social work has yet to develop a significant anti-poverty perspective (Becker, 1997).

Thus, the desire of the social work profession to distance itself from its 19th-century roots has resulted in a somewhat ambiguous relationship between the profession and cash payments to those in need. Against this background, the introduction of direct payments in 1996 must be seen as a radical departure from current social work practice, re-establishing the profession's links to its pre-1948 history. Although direct payments are provided in lieu of services and are therefore very different from outdoor relief or COS charity, the involvement of social workers in making cash payments to disabled people represents a fundamental shift in the nature of the profession, turning the clock back nearly 50 years. This is not only of interest to the social historian and to social work academics, but may also help to explain why many social services departments have been slow to take up the opportunities offered by direct payments (see Chapters Three to Five and Eight).

Certainly, concerns about a potential shift in social work practice were prominent in the early 1990s following a number of attempts to introduce a private member's bill to legalise direct payments (see Chapter Three). In response, the health secretary, Virginia Bottomley, wrote to the MP responsible suggesting that "social services legislation is concerned with the arrangements of services and not with direct payments, which is the province of the social security system" (quoted in Hatchett, 1991, pp 14-15). Several years later, the issue was to re-emerge following the passage of the 1996 Community Care (Direct Payments) Act, with fears that social services departments might be turned into 'income maintenance organisations' and that the Benefits Agency may be considering transferring the administration of certain disability benefits to social services (Hirst, 1997). Although these fears proved groundless, they demonstrated the fundamental shift that was taking place within social work practice as a result of the introduction of direct payments and provided an early indication that the social work profession might not necessarily welcome the new reforms with open arms (see Chapters Five and Eight for further details).

Pressure for direct payments

Following the introduction of the 1948 National Assistance Act, service provision has begun to evolve away from its initial emphasis on residential care to include a much wider range of community services (Means and Smith, 1998a, b). Despite this, pressure for change and for more responsive and flexible services has increased, culminating in 1996 with the passage of the Community Care (Direct Payments) Act to enable certain groups of service users to receive cash payments with which to purchase their own care. Although there is still relatively little literature in this area, research has suggested that the introduction of direct payments can be traced to three separate but inter-related developments (Glendinning et al, 2000a, pp 7-9):

- the shortcomings of directly provided services;
- pressure from the Independent Living Movement;
- the experience of the Independent Living Fund;

As a result, the remainder of this chapter reviews each of these developments in turn.

Directly provided services

Following the community care reforms of the 1990s, there is increasing evidence that services provided directly by local authority social services department are too inflexible and unresponsive to meet the needs of many service users. In 1994, the British Council of Disabled People (BCODP) published the results of research based on interviews with 70 disabled people from four case study local authorities in the Midlands, the South of England and Inner and Outer London (Zarb and Nadash, 1994). Although the findings of this study are discussed in further detail in Chapters Three, Five and Seven, the research highlighted a number of disadvantages within existing social services (see Box 2). While some people felt that directly provided services had a number of advantages, common criticisms included: lack of control, lack of flexibility, and lack of reliability of such services (Zarb and Nadash, 1994, ch 6).

After the full implementation of the NHS and Community Care Act in 1993, social services departments were given a specific brief to target scarce resources on those with the greatest needs (DoH, 1990). With regard to domiciliary care, this has accelerated the trend towards rebranding traditional 'home help' services as 'home care', focusing on personal care rather than housework and often excluding people with 'low level' needs (Clark et al, 1998). Frequently such changes are accompanied by an increased tendency to define home care interventions in terms of specific tasks, rather than on an hourly basis, leading to complaints of institutionalisation and of reducing opportunities for more generalised social interaction between carers and service users (Glendinning et al, 2000a). At the same time, reductions in the length of hospital stays and the emphasis on maximising the throughput of patients have

Box 2: Disadvantages of directly provided services

1 **Lack of control over times support is supplied**:
- Disrupts day-to-day routines
- Reduces personal freedom
- Unreliable

2 **Lack of control over who provides assistance**:
- Increases feelings of intrusion on privacy
- Reduces choice over characteristics of support workers (for example, age and gender)
- No sanctions to ensure quality of assistance provided (other than complaints procedures adopted by service providers)

3 **Inability to control type of assistance and how it is provided**:
- Leads to inefficiency (for example, workers breaking things, putting household items away in the wrong place, not preparing food to personal tastes)
- Increases stress
- Reduces personal dignity and feeling of being in control of one's life

4 **Unreliability**:
- Increases stress and practical inconvenience
- Reduces ability to control times when assistance is provided
- Can disrupt family life, social life and other activities
- Sanctions available limited if services do not respond to requests for support
- Reduces confidence in support arrangements
- Increases practical demands on other family members

5 **Lack of flexibility**:
- Can create gaps in assistance provided
- Reduces likelihood of securing back-up and emergency cover for usual sources of support
- Reduces ability to increase support when needs vary
- Can increase vulnerability to breakdown of support arrangements
- Increases reliance on respite services
- Increases reliance on informal support

6 **Interpersonal relationships with staff**:
- Lack of choice over staff can lead to intrusion on privacy
- Difficulties with changing staff if interpersonal problems arise
- Limited sanctions available if unhappy with attitudes or behaviour of staff
- Larger number of staff to deal with can be inconvenient and/or stressful

7 **Other disadvantages**:
- Increased vulnerability if service provision reduced or withdrawn
- Uncertainty about future levels of local community care provision
- Concerns about charging and/or means testing

(Zarb and Nadash, 1994, pp 88-90)

resulted in patients being discharged to the community with far greater health needs than would once have been the case (Glasby and Littlechild, 2000a, b). This has meant that district nurses are dealing with increasingly complex needs and focusing much more on technical nursing care, leaving users with fewer health needs to social services home carers (Barret and Hudson, 1997). Throughout all these changes, there is a growing consensus that care remains service- rather than needs-led, and that both health and social care providers are geared more to crisis intervention than to promoting independence and social inclusion (Morris, 1993a; Glasby and Littlechild, 2000a).

Perhaps the most striking examples of the inflexibility of traditional services comes from Morris' (1993a) description of the experiences of fifty disabled people aged between 19 and 55. This research paints a distressing picture of restrictive services that seek to fit the individual to the service and serve only to enhance, rather than reduce, dependency (see Box 3). Against this background, direct payments must be seen as a means of enhancing both choice and control, overcoming the traditional limitations of directly provided services.

Independent living

Although the shortcomings of directly provided community care services are widely recognised, the most vehement criticisms have often come from the

Box 3: Fitting the individual to the service

Marcia's home carers will not assist her with housework or shopping.

Home carers would not assist Mary's husband to have a bath, and the family had to approach their GP to argue that Mary's husband needed a bath for medical reasons.

To get help washing his clothes, William had to argue that this need was created by incontinence.

Catherine's social services department offered to send someone round between 5 and 7 o'clock as this was when they had staff available – even though Catherine did not need assistance at this time.

Elizabeth is Afro-Caribbean and feels that white home carers do not know how to look after her hair properly.

One carer argued with Susan about the way her underwear was placed. Susan tried to deal with this politely, but eventually lost her temper: "Who's fucking wearing it, me or you?"

Vicky feels that the care assistants who visit her are homophobic and do not understand her life. (Morris, 1993a, ch 7)

Independent Living Movement. The concept of independent living originated in 1973 in the US, where three disabled students were able to attend university at Berkeley, California with the support of personal assistants (PAs) provided by the university (Evans, 1993). After graduation, these three students felt that the PA system had been so successful that they established the world's first Centre for Independent Living (CIL), an organisation run and controlled by disabled people which sought to support other disabled people in taking greater control of their lives and services. Nicknamed the 'quad squad' (since most of the original students were paralysed from the shoulders down), one of the students used an iron lung and went on to become the equivalent of the Director of Social Services in California (Evans, 1993, p 59). Initially, the Berkley CIL had five key aims, focusing on housing, personal assistance, accessible transport, an accessible environment and peer support. Within 10 years, there were 200 CILs in America (Evans, 1993, p 60), and the concept began to spread overseas. In the UK, CILs were founded in Hampshire and in Derbyshire during the early 1980s. Also at this time, the formation of the BCODP (established in 1981) and the European Network on Integrated Living (ENIL) (established in 1989) provided national and international forums for the promotion of independent living (Morris, 1993a). More recently, the creation of a National Centre for Independent Living (NCIL) (a BCODP project) has served to act as a further focus for the Independent Living Movement. From the beginning, the concept of PAs working under the control of disabled people has been a central feature of independent living, pioneering many of the concepts which were later to form part of the direct payments introduced in Britain in 1996 (Zarb and Nadash, 1994, p 5).

The philosophy of the Independent Living Movement is based on four key assumptions (Morris, 1993a, p 21):

- All human life is of value.
- Anyone, whatever their impairment, is capable of exercising choices.
- People who are disabled by society's reaction to physical, intellectual and sensory impairment and to emotional distress have the right to assert control over their lives.
- Disabled people have the right to participate fully in society.

Although definitions of independent living vary, they all emphasise the importance of choice and control (see Box 4) – central features of the 1996 Community Care (Direct Payments) Act. Indeed, disabled activists such as Frances Hasler are adamant that direct payments are only a means to achieving the overall goal of independent living (Hasler, 2000, p 6):

> Direct payments are a means to an end and that end is independent living. We need to hang on to that. Direct payments are not a good thing or a bad thing in themselves. Direct payments are just a way of getting to independent living.

Box 4: Independent living

Independent living is the concept of the empowerment of disabled people and their ability to control their own lives.

Independent living is when disabled people live within the community and control the decisions affecting their own lives.

Independent living is a way of choosing and taking control of your own lifestyle. It is all about choosing and controlling what to do, when to do it, and who should do it.

Independent living is a dynamic process. It is about creating choices and identifying solutions. It is a way of life that grows as you grow and develops as you develop.

Independent living is a philosophy and a movement of disabled people who work for equal rights and equal opportunities, self-respect and self-determination. Independent living does not mean that disabled people do not need anybody, that they want to do everything by themselves in isolation. Independent living means that disabled people want the same life opportunities and the same choices in every day life that their non-disabled brothers and sisters, neighbours and friends take for granted. That includes growing up in their families, going to the neighbourhood school, using the same bus, getting employment that is in line with their education and abilities, having equal access to the same services and establishments of social life, culture and leisure. Most importantly, just like everyone else, disabled people need to be in charge of their own lives, need to think and speak for themselves without interference from others.... In order to reach the same control and the same choices in every day life that non-disabled persons take for granted a number of prerequisites are necessary. For persons with extensive disabilities there are two key requirements: personal assistance and accessibility in the built environment including accessible housing. Without these two necessities persons with extensive disabilities, in many countries, can only choose between being a burden on their families or living in an institution. These extremely limited and limiting options are incompatible with the concept of independent living.

(NCIL, nda; Ratzka, nd)

The Independent Living Fund

Prior to the introduction of direct payments, the Independent Living Fund (ILF) gave disabled people the opportunity to receive cash payments in order to purchase personal assistance. In 1986, the Social Security Act announced measures to replace Supplementary Benefit with Income Support. Whereas recipients of Supplementary Benefit could receive additional payments on the basis of ill-health or disability, the new Income Support would replace such additions with flat rate disability and severe disability premiums, with much stricter eligibility criteria than the previous system (Hudson, 1988, 1994).

Contemporary estimates suggested that some disabled people could be as much as £50 per week worse off as a result of these changes, and that some of these people would be forced into residential care (Hudson, 1988; Kestenbaum, 1993a).

In response, disability groups began a sustained lobbying process, eventually succeeding in persuading the then Conservative government to make alternative arrangements for those affected by the 1986 Act. After consulting with representatives of disability groups, Nicholas Scott, Minister for Social Security and the Disabled, announced details of a new ILF in early 1988 (Kestenbaum, 1993a). The ILF was to be an independent trust fund with half the trustees nominated by the then Department of Health and Social Security and half nominated by the DIG. Established for a maximum of five years with an initial budget of £5 million, the ILF would make payments to a small number of disabled people who had to pay for personal assistance. The number of applicants was expected to be "in the hundreds rather than the thousands" (quoted in Hudson, 1988, p 708), and the Fund was only available to those disabled people on low incomes who had to pay for personal care.

From the beginning, it quickly became apparent that the government had significantly underestimated the demand for the ILF. Although it was initially anticipated that there would be around 300 new awards each year, applications reached the rate of 900 per month in 1989-90 and, by November 1992, 2000 per month (Kestenbaum, 1993a, pp 29-33). By 1993, some 22,000 people were receiving payments (Zarb and Nadash, 1994, p 6) and the fund had an annual budget of £82 million (Kestenbaum, 1993a, p 32). Research carried out by the ILF suggested that the popularity of this new form of support was largely due to the enhanced choice and control which it enabled (see Box 5). Drawing on semi-structured interviews with ILF recipients and a large-scale postal questionnaire, the ILF research officer found that the most valued aspects of receiving cash to purchase care included (Kestenbaum, 1993b, pp 32-41):

- choice of care assistant;
- continuity of care;
- the flexibility of care arrangements;
- the greater availability of respite options;
- enhanced self-respect;
- control.

As Kestenbaum has demonstrated:

> For many applicants, the ILF was not just about making up for unavailable statutory services. It was the preferred option. From a disabled person's point of view, the provision of cash makes the important difference between having one's personal life controlled by others and exercising choices and control for oneself. Money has enabled ILF clients ... not only to avoid going into residential care, but also to determine for themselves the help they require and how and when they want it to be provided. (1993a, p 35)

> The findings from this research challenge the assumption that disabled people are incapable of exercising effective choice and control over their own care arrangements.... The experience of ILF clients ... shows how, with enough money to have care assistance under their own control, or that of a chosen advocate, many disabled people can greatly improve the quality of their lives as well as stay out of residential care. (1993b, p 78)

Perhaps inevitably, the success of the ILF posed both financial and political problems for the government (Morris, 1993a, p 14). While the Fund had uncovered the need for cash payments to enable disabled people to purchase their own care, the cost was escalating rapidly and local authorities (the lead agencies under the community reforms introduced in 1993) were prohibited from making such payments (see Chapter Three for further details). After tightening eligibility criteria in 1990 and 1992 and introducing an age limit on the Fund (excluding those aged 75 and over), the ultimate response of the government was to terminate the original ILF, and to replace it with two successor bodies (Hudson, 1993; ILF, 2000):

- The Independent Living (Extension) Fund would continue to administer payments to recipients of the original ILF, although awards are not linked to inflation.
- The Independent Living (1993) Fund would accept new applications but on a different basis. Henceforth, disabled people receiving at least £200 worth of services per week from their local authority may receive a maximum of £375 from the Fund. Crucially, the new Fund was to be restricted to people aged under 66 at the time of their application (see Kestenbaum, 1999, appendix A and ILF, 2000 for eligibility criteria).

Box 5: Users' experiences of the Independent Living Fund

"If you're paying for it you can get what you want."

"You can do what you want when you want to do it."

"Having the cash to pay for the things you need means that you have standing. You're more in control of your life. That's what you're trying to achieve all the time."

"Having the cash means you aren't always on the receiving end. You feel better having two way traffic – give and take."

"I think this is the best way. You're in charge of your own destiny. We're the boss, aren't we?"

(Kestenbaum, 1993b, pp 35-8; see also Lakey, 1994)

Thus, from April 1993, local authority social services departments were responsible for purchasing services to meet the assessed needs of disabled people, using the new ILF to 'top up' existing care packages. This was widely interpreted as a retrograde step which emphasised professional control rather than user-led services and independent living, and the 1993 changes were greeted with widespread dissatisfaction (see, for example, Hudson, 1993; Morris, 1993b). Despite this, the experience of the ILF did reveal a number of significant issues that were later to influence the initial introduction and subsequent expansion of direct payments.

On a practical level, the experience of using ILF payments raised several issues that were later to be revisited after the implementation of direct payments:

- A number of prominent cases raised the need for adequate support systems to ensure that disabled people purchasing their own care were able to meet their legal and financial obligations (see Chapter Nine). In some cases, ILF recipients were left in thousands of pounds worth of debt having failed to make National Insurance and other contributions, serving as a powerful reminder of the need to focus on the technicalities of being an employer (Bond, 1996).
- Some disabled people can find it very difficult to recruit PAs, and may value support in this area (Kestenbaum, 1993b, pp 12-13).
- At the same time, concerns were expressed that any payments to disabled people should take additional costs such as recruitment, employers' contributions and other overheads fully into account (Bond, 1996).
- Some ILF recipients were nervous about what would happen when the community care reforms were introduced and feared that they could lose their payments (Kestenbaum, 1993b, p 41). During the late 1990s, similar issues were to be raised following the tendency of many local authorities to introduce direct payments on a pilot basis, leaving some service users unsure as to whether or not pilot projects would become part of mainstream service provision (see Chapters Three and Five).
- The ILF revealed the potential conflicts which can arise between the aims of the Independent Living Movement and the desire of central government to limit public expenditure (see Chapter Eight for further details).

Above all, however, the ILF enabled disabled people to purchase their own care and represented a fundamental shift in power between professionals and users. As Hudson has commented:

> The ILF offered precisely what many people wanted – a major weekly cash payment ... direct to claimants to buy the support they felt they required. For the first time in Britain, users were calling the shots in the purchase and provision of care.... In a major and unintended way, the 1986 Social Security Act produced a visionary glimpse of the reality and feasibility of user-led care packages. (1993, p 28)

This was not the original aim of the government, and Morris (1993a, p 13) uses the phrase "progress by default" to describe how a small-scale government policy measure could have such significant implications for the Independent Living Movement. With hindsight, however, the ILF must be seen as a 'Pandora's box' (Hudson, 1993, p 28) which, once opened, would be very difficult to close again.

SUMMARY

In order to overcome the stigma of the Poor Law, postwar social work in Britain has been characterised by the separation of social security and social services, with the former focusing on financial needs and the latter on providing welfare services for frail and disabled people. Once widely hailed as a step forward, this separation has since been criticised for enforcing an artificial distinction which does not adequately reflect people's needs, and for depriving social work of an awareness of poverty issues. Against this background, the decision to enable local authorities to make cash payments in lieu of directly provided services represents a major cultural shift that significantly alters the role of social services departments. As a result, those seeking to promote direct payments need to be aware of the magnitude of the task ahead of them in seeking to overcome social workers' opposition to this new way of working (see Chapter Eight for further discussion).

Prior to the introduction of direct payments in 1996, pressure for reform had been mounting for some time. Crucially, key figures in the campaign for change were disabled people themselves, critiquing local authority services, organising themselves into an Independent Living Movement and persuading the government to introduce the ILF. As criticisms of directly provided services increased, the experience of receiving ILF payments began to alter the relationship between service users and service providers, demonstrating the liberating and empowering potential of disabled people purchasing personal assistance directly. Although the government acted in order to limit the scope of the ILF, services could not return to the pre-1988 situation and reform of some description was almost inevitable.

THREE

From indirect to direct payments I: legislation

Despite the growth of the Independent Living Movement and the popularity of the ILF, direct payments to individual service users were illegal until the passage of the 1996 Community Care (Direct Payments) Act. This was the result of a desire to separate social work from its 19th-century roots (see Chapter Two) and was embodied in three main statutes (Mandelstam, 1999, p 232):

- Section 29 of the 1948 National Assistance Act (see Box 6);
- Section 45 of the 1968 Health Service and Public Health Act;
- Schedule 8 of the 1977 National Health Service Act.

Although the 1968 Social Work (Scotland) Act did permit direct payments in certain circumstances, these were heavily prescribed and the power to make such payments was rarely used (Zarb and Nadash, 1994; Witcher et al, 2000; see Chapter Five for further details).

Despite these legal obstacles, we have already seen how pressure had begun to build for some sort of cash payment to enable disabled people to make their own care arrangements (Chapter Two). As this pressure continued to mount, key milestones in the eventual introduction of direct payments included:

- the growth of indirect payments in the 1980s and 1990s, whereby disabled people established their own trusts to administer cash payments, or where money was paid via third parties;
- thwarted attempts to introduce direct payments in the early 1990s;
- the 1996 Community Care (Direct Payments) Act;
- official policy and practice guidance;
- the subsequent extension of direct payments to different user groups.

Box 6: Direct payments prior to 1996

Nothing in the foregoing provisions of this section shall authorise or require – a) the payment of money to persons to whom this section applies ... [that is to say persons who are blind, deaf or dumb, and other persons who are substantially and permanently handicapped by illness, injury, or congenital deformity.]

(1948 National Assistance Act, section 29)

While events leading up to the passage of the 1996 Community Care (Direct Payments) Act are examined in this chapter, official guidance and subsequent developments are explored in Chapter Four.

Indirect payments

As awareness about the potential advantages of enabling disabled people to purchase their own care increased, both service users and local authorities began to explore methods of circumventing the prohibitions of the National Assistance Act. For John Evans, then chair of the BCODP Independent Living committee, it was crucial to get rid of "that damn silly law from 1948, and accept that direct payments for some people are just common sense" (quoted in George, 1994a, p 15). Others agreed, and a range of schemes were developed in different parts of the country to make payments to disabled people, some of them of doubtful legality (Mandelstam, 1999). Although arrangements varied, the two main approaches were to make payments via a third party (such as a voluntary agency) or via an independent trust (see Boxes 7 and 8).

Probably the first example of indirect payments was in Hampshire in the early 1980s, where a group of disabled people were able to move out of residential care after persuading their local authority to take the pioneering step of making payments to each individual via the original residential home (Project 81, nd; Shearer, 1984; Zarb and Nadash, 1994, pp 5-6). Although the Hampshire scheme faced closure because of legal concerns raised by the county's solicitor and treasurer, a report from the Audit Commission (1986, p 69) specifically cited Hampshire's payment scheme as an example of innovative good practice (Evans and Hasler, 1996). This proved enough to save the scheme, and Hampshire has remained a key player during the implementation of direct payments (see Chapter Five).

Since then, payment schemes began to expand and, in 1990, research commissioned by RADAR[1] found that 59% of 69 participating local authorities made payments to disabled people, either directly or indirectly through intermediaries (quoted in Hatchett, 1991, p 14). The latter included charities, housing associations and national organisations such as the Spinal Injuries Association (Hatchett, 1991, p 14; Craig, 1992, p 47; Morris, 1993a, p 26). Although payment recipients were often individuals who had taken the initiative in putting their case to the local authority (Morris, 1993a), most participating authorities in the study suggested that they would welcome legislation enabling them to make such payments (Craig, 1992, p 47).

In 1994, researchers from the Policy Studies Institute (PSI) carried out a national postal survey of local authorities in England, Wales and Scotland, with a 64% response rate (Zarb and Nadash, 1994). The study found that just under 60% of participating authorities were already operating payments schemes (most of which involved indirect payments through a third party or through trusts). This figure was almost identical to the RADAR study of 1990, the key difference being that there was far less evidence in the 1994 survey of authorities making payments directly to service users than in 1990 (5% and 23% respectively).

However, this was felt to be a product of contemporary legal concerns, following government statements on the illegality of direct payments (to be discussed later). As a result, several authorities had taken legal advice, changed from direct to indirect payments or ceased making payments altogether. Despite this, just over 90% of respondents indicated that they would make direct payments if legislation permitted, with only three authorities stating that they were definitely opposed to such changes.

Box 7: Indirect payments

To overcome legal restrictions, Lauren used to receive payments from her local authority via a housing association. This meant that the housing association was the employer, not Lauren. So she took further action to enhance her control of her care package. On the suggestion of a friend, Lauren set up a trust to receive the payments on her behalf. The trust deed was drawn up by a solicitor, and Lauren served as a trustee together with three friends. Lauren now employs four PAs and is able to work and care for her mother. To ensure accountability to the local authority, a social worker sits on the trust. (Morris, 1993a, p 122)

A local authority can set up a non-charitable Trust for the benefit of an individual. This means that the local authority hands an agreed sum of money over each year to a Trust which is set up for the benefit of an individual or individuals. In the case of one individual, there are usually three or four trustees, of whom the individual (the 'Principal Beneficiary') is one and the day-to-day management of the Trust is delegated to this person. The other trustees can be friends, a solicitor, an accountant or anyone else who you think would be useful to you. (Morris, 1995)

There are examples of severely disabled people living in the community. One of the best is provided by the Centre for Independent Living based at Lee Court Cheshire Home in Hampshire. The Social Services Department and Health Authority have contributed funds to a trust for purchasing care which is administered by the Leonard Cheshire Foundation. The disabled person buys in the help they need with this money, topped up by his or her own social security benefits. Thus the disabled people construct their own packages of care and employ their own staff in a highly autonomous fashion. (Audit Commission, 1986, p 69)

One example [of indirect payments via a third party] is that of Lothian Social Work Department who, having assessed someone's personal assistance needs, makes a quarterly cash payment in advance for the cost of paying for that assistance to the Edinburgh Voluntary Organisation Council. The payment is passed on to the individual who then uses it to either employ their own personal assistants, or to employ agency staff. (Morris, 1995)

Further information about the very influential Kingston scheme is provided in Chapter Four (see also Macfarlane, 1990 and Webb, 1996).

Box 8: Indirect payments in Norfolk

With funding from the local social services department and the Joseph Rowntree Foundation, Norfolk's Independent Living Project (ILP) was launched in 1993 to enable disabled people to live independently in the community and provide support for people employing their own PAs. Working in partnership with a number of voluntary agencies, the social services department was unable to pay money directly to disabled service users, but could make indirect payments via the ILP. (Dawson, 2000)

Thwarted reforms

As evidence of the benefits of paying cash sums to individual service users increased, so pressure began to mount for legislation to legalise direct payments. Throughout this process, organisations of disabled people and advocates of independent living have been at the forefront of the campaign for change, lobbying Members of Parliament, organising meetings and commissioning research (see Box 9). A good example of the way in which disabled people were able to take the lead in the campaign for direct payments comes from Kingston-upon-Thames, where an early and prominent payments scheme was established on the initiative of two local disabled people (to be discussed later). As part of this process, the disabled people approached the social services department with their proposal for a payments scheme, produced formal documentation for the social services committee and participated in a pilot scheme (Macfarlane, 1990; DoH, 1998c).

As part of the lobbying process, BCODP quickly found an influential supporter in Andrew Rowe, Conservative MP for Faversham and mid-Kent (Evans and Hasler, 1996). Having encountered the concept of direct payments

Box 9: The campaign for direct payments

The Direct Payments scheme in the UK was started in 1989 by the BCODP IL [Independent Living] Committee.... In the early 1990s ... BCODP ... got together with the Spinal Injuries Association and its parliamentary officer Fidelity Simpson who was an expert in lobbying tactics and parliamentary affairs. This group then drew up a tactical strategy for bringing about Direct Payments legislation. Key disabled people from both these organisations with direct experience of running their own schemes worked together with Fidelity targeting possible key allies of members of Parliament and politicians who would support and fight our cause. Many letters were written to local and national politicians seeking support. Numerous awareness-raising campaigns and briefing meetings were arranged, and relevant publicity was drawn up to disseminate information in order to make the issue public and clear, together with articles in both the mainstream and disability press. (Evans and Hasler, 1996) through a disabled member of his constituency, Rowe became a committed supporter of the Independent Living Movement and was a key player in campaigning for the legislative changes which were finally to be introduced under the 1996 Community Care (Direct Payments) Act. During parliamentary debates on the NHS and Community Care Bill in 1990, Rowe raised the issue of direct payments in front of a House of Commons Standing Committee and proposed an amendment to the Bill permitting such payments to be made (see Box 10). In response, the Secretary of State for Health, Virginia Bottomley, admitted the logic of direct payments, signalled the government's commitment to such an amendment and promised to consider Andrew Rowe's proposal in more detail (SC(E), 22/02/1990, cols 1229-30). When no response appeared to be forthcoming, Andrew Rowe's attempts to promote direct payments were taken up in the House of Lords by Baroness Masham of Ilton, who sought unsuccessfully to introduce a similar amendment to the NHS and Community Care Bill (see Box 10). Like Andrew Rowe's initial amendment, this clause was withdrawn on the grounds that the government would consider the proposal with a view to amending the NHS and Community Care Bill (HLD 10/05/1990 col 1589).

Unfortunately, this action was to backfire, with serious and unintended consequences. Having examined the issue of making cash payments to disabled people, the government found that this practice was illegal under the 1948 National Assistance Act and took action to remind local authorities of their statutory responsibilities through policy guidance accompanying the community

Box 10: Direct payments and the NHS and Community Care Bill

House of Commons: New Clause 3

Disabled Persons (Care or Assistance Services)

Notwithstanding the provisions of section 29(6) of the National Assistance Act 1948, a local authority shall be authorised to make payments to a disabled person for the purchase of care or personal assistance services. (SC(E), 22/02/1990 col 1223)

House of Lords: Amendment No 115ZC

After Clause 45, insert the following new clause:

Payments for the purchase of care or personal assistance

Notwithstanding the provisions of section 29(6) of the National Assistance Act 1948, a local authority, having regard to any guidance issued by the Secretary of State, may make payments to a disabled person for the purchase of care or personal assistance services. (HLD 10/05/1990 col 1589)

Box 11: Prohibition of direct payments

It may be possible for some service users to play a more active part in their own care management, for example assuming responsibility for the day-to-day management of their carers may help to meet the aspirations of severely physically disabled people to be as independent as possible. In these circumstances systems of accountability will have to be clearly defined. Authorities are reminded that Section 29 of the 1948 Act and Schedule 8 to the 1977 Act, as well as Section 45 of the 1968 Act, prohibit the making of cash payments in place of arranging services. (DoH, 1990, p 26)

care reforms (see Box 11). Thus, a measure designed to promote the concept of direct payments and support existing payment schemes, had actually resulted in such schemes being declared illegal (personal communication, Andrew Rowe). This was to cause considerable difficulties for a number of local authorities, who were broadly supportive of direct payments yet were understandably concerned to be seen to be operating within the law.

Once direct payments had been declared illegal, the only course of action was to campaign for new legislation to overturn this prohibition. In 1992, Andrew Rowe sought to atone for his earlier intervention by introducing a Private Members' Bill on direct payments. Under the Disabled Persons (Services) Bill, disabled people, who were able and willing, would be permitted to employ their own staff with the bills paid by the local authority (see Box 12). While Andrew Rowe's preferred choice was for disabled people to control their own payments, his Bill was designed to overcome considerable Treasury concerns about the danger of public money being misappropriated (personal communication). Although the Bill was defeated, it was introduced in the House of Lords on 30 March 1993 by Lord McColl (see Box 13) in the form of the Disabled Persons (Services) (No 2) Bill (HLD, 30/03/1993, cols 724-5). Although this Bill did rather better than its predecessor, it too failed to become legislation.

Box 12: The Disabled Persons (Services) Bill

I propose that such disabled people as are assessed as able and willing to shoulder the responsibility of recruiting and employing their own staff should be allowed to do so up to the financial limit decreed by the local authority. They should then arrange to have the bills paid by the local authority, but the responsibility for the staff contracts would be theirs.... The Bill is modest, but the principle that it enshrines is fundamental to community care. Community care is partly about enhancing the dignity of those who need public care. It is also about enhancing choice, developing personal responsibility and encouraging the growth of personal capacity. It must, therefore, be right to allow those disabled people who have the capacity and the desire to take control of the most personal part of the care arrangements to do so. (HCD, 24/06/1992, col 267)

Box 13: The Disabled Person's (Services) (No 2) Bill

An Act to empower local authorities to make certain severely disabled persons accountable for expenditure on their care plans.
...The duty of a local authority to make welfare arrangements [for disabled people] ... may be discharged by the making of an allowance paid directly to a disabled person ..., provided that the total of payments to any person under this section does not exceed the total of expenditure for the same purposes which may be made in this respect of that person under any other enactment.
A person covered by this subsection must ... have signified to the local authority concerned his consent in writing.

During the various parliamentary debates which accompanied these events, the arguments for and against direct payments emerged time and time again (based on Zarb and Nadash, 1994, pp 9–11):

Advantages of direct payments

- providing disabled people with choice and control;
- enhancing dignity and privacy;
- reducing dependence on informal carers;
- cost-efficiency (providing high quality support at low costs);
- consistent with the emphasis of the community care reforms on choice and user involvement;
- supported by a wide range of disability and professional groups.

Disadvantages of direct payments

- the complexity of administering direct payments and doubts about the capacity of local authorities to manage payment schemes;
- the community care reforms would extend choice and control without the need for direct payments;
- concerns that direct payments would reduce local authorities' flexibility in providing services and divert resources from other priorities;
- fears that direct payments would 'open the floodgates' by creating an unknown and potentially unlimited level of demand.

Other concerns about direct payments included the perceived difficulty of establishing adequate procedures to ensure that public money was spent appropriately and the possible risk that PAs might exploit or abuse disabled people (see Zarb and Nadash, 1994; Campbell, 1996).

Throughout the events described above, considerable lobbying and campaigning was taking place, without much apparent success. While groups of disabled people met key politicians on a number of occasions (see Box 14), supporters such as Andrew Rowe describe how frustratingly slow the

Box 14: Slow progress

During this time when Andrew Rowe was trying to progress his Direct Payments Bill, the campaign group organised a number of meetings with key politicians to try and influence them about the issue. These included the then current Minister of Health, and the Minister for disabled people. Both of these politicians expressed how much they appreciated independent living schemes, but neither were prepared to take serious action and publicly support them. Our understanding of the situation then was that the treasury department was not in support of this kind of legislation because of the economic argument of it costing too much. These developments exasperated the campaign group and the Independent Living movement. (Evans and Hasler, 1996)

government's responses were (personal communication). In response, the BCODP Independent Living Committee decided to change its tactics somewhat, commissioning independent research in order to investigate the cost implications and effectiveness of direct payment schemes. With funding from the Joseph Rowntree Foundation, BCODP were able to commission the PSI to undertake the desired research. The resulting study, *Cashing in on independence* (Zarb and Nadash, 1994), was a seminal document and is referred to time and time again throughout this book. While it is difficult to gauge how successful it was in persuading the government to implement direct payments, it must undoubtedly have been a factor in the government's eventual change of heart on the direct payments issue (to be discussed later).

Despite government opposition to direct payments and the defeat of Andrew Rowe's proposed legislation, the BCODP campaign did receive significant support from other bodies, most notably from the Association of Directors of Social Services (ADSS) (Evans and Hasler, 1996). In 1992, the ADSS adopted a resolution in support of direct payments (see Box 15) and became an increasingly active member of the campaign for a change in the law. In addition to writing the foreword to *Cashing in on independence* (Zarb and Nadash, 1994), Roy Taylor (then chair of the ADSS Disabilities Committee) was a key player in the struggle for direct payments (see, for example, Taylor, 1994, 1995, 1996a, 1996b, 1997) and a substantial body of material from this period has been maintained in the form of a mini-archive. In addition to the ADSS, other key supporters of direct payments included the Audit Commission, the Prince of Wales Advisory Group on Disability and the British Association of Social Workers (HLD, 21/04/1993, col 1642), as well as the Association of Metropolitan Authorities (Evans, 2000). Also at this time, the concept of direct payments received qualified support from the House of Commons Select Committee on Health, which felt that more research was required before direct payments could be implemented, but that such payments were consistent with the emphasis of the community care reforms on user involvement and enhancing choice (House of Commons Health Committee, 1993, pp xv-xvi).

Box 15: Direct payments and the ADSS

This association requests that local authorities be empowered, following an assessment of need, to make direct payments to disabled people in order that they can buy and organise their own services, allowing personal autonomy and control. (quoted in Taylor, 1996a)

Throughout the campaign for direct payments, uncertainty about what the future may hold was undoubtedly a major concern for many disabled people. With the legality of payment schemes thrown into doubt and a series of abortive attempts to introduce new legislation, many disabled people were unsure about the future availability of payments (Zarb and Nadash, 1994). This uncertainty was later to continue after the implementation of the 1996 Community Care (Direct Payments) Act, for the discretionary nature of the reforms meant that disabled people had no guarantees that the various direct payment schemes which were initially piloted would continue and be adopted into mainstream service provision (see Chapter Five). In many ways, this was similar to events in the early 1990s, when the introduction of the community care reforms led to fears about the future availability of ILF payments (see Chapter Two).

The 1996 Community Care (Direct Payments) Act

In November 1994, the government announced its intention to legislate in order to enable local authorities to make direct payments to service users rather than providing community care services directly:

> I [Virginia Bottomley, Health Secretary] intend to take, in conjunction with my Rt. Hon. Friends the Secretaries of State for Scotland and Wales, a new power to enable social services authorities and social work departments to make direct cash payments to disabled people in lieu of community care services. Direct payments ... will give disabled people greater independence and choice and involve them and their carers more fully in their own care. (DoH, 1994, p 1)

While it may never be entirely clear what factors were responsible for this change of heart, there appear to have been a number of key considerations. As Box 16 suggests, the imminent launch of the BCODP/PSI research into direct payments may have been a key factor in persuading the government to reconsider its previous opposition to direct payments. For Andrew Rowe, direct payments were the result of a dedicated and sustained campaign for reform and the momentum for change was simply too strong for the government to resist. Ultimately, "Direct payments were an idea whose time had long since come" (Andrew Rowe, personal communication).

Box 16: A government change of heart

Interestingly enough, a week before the BCODP/PSI launch of the Direct Payment research findings, called 'Cashing in on Independence', the Minister of Health announced that it was the Government's intention to bring about Direct Payments legislation in the next parliamentary year. We were ecstatic! After five years of campaigning vigorously, we had achieved the beginning of our main goal. This announcement led to an intense flurry of activity around the whole issue of Direct Payments and a proliferation of seminars and conferences were organised by both policy makers and the Independent Living movement. Also, numerous research projects on independent living issues were instigated. At one of these conferences organised by the SSI, the Social Services Inspectorate, a number of independent living advocates met up with some key civil servants, who had been delegated the task by the Department of Health to research and work on implementing the Direct Payments change. From now on they were crucial in our deliberations and strategies. (Evans and Hasler, 1996)

Once the decision had been taken to introduce direct payments, a number of practical matters needed to be resolved before new legislation could be drawn up. As a result, a Technical Advisory Group (TAG) met to consider some of the technical issues which implementation would raise (see Box 17). Including representatives from central government, local authorities and organisations of disabled people, TAG examined some of the key issues that direct payments would raise, drew up guidance for government ministers and civil servants and contributed to the 1996 consultation paper on direct payments (see Box 18 and discussion on page 29). Although the group included three disability organisations, only one member of TAG was a personal assistance user running her own direct payment scheme (Evans and Hasler, 1996).

Building on the work of TAG, the Department of Health introduced a consultation paper in January 1996 on its proposals for direct payments (DoH/Scottish Office/Welsh Office/Northern Ireland Office, 1996). In addition to setting out how direct payments would operate, the consultation paper sought views on a number of key issues to be contained within the regulations and guidance. Central to the government's view of how direct payments should function was the belief that recipients must be 'willing' to receive payments instead of services and 'able' to manage them (DoH/Scottish Office/Welsh Office/Northern Ireland Office, 1996, p 3). While service users could receive extensive support from others, they would ultimately remain responsible for the management of their payments.

Crucially, the Direct Payments Bill would give the Secretary of State the power to specify which groups of people could receive direct payments, a move justified in terms of the need to restrict the number of direct payment recipients while the scheme was in its infancy (see Box 18). As a result, the consultation paper set out six possible groups of people that may be able to benefit from direct payments, emphasising that its own preference was to limit direct payments to the first group only (that is, to people with physical

Box 17: The Technical Advisory Group

Margaret Baldwin	Independent Living Fund
Jane Campbell	British Council of Disabled People
Gary Flather QC	Chairman of the Bar Council Disability Panel
John Keep	Royal Association for Disability and Rehabilitation
Vivien Lawson	Social Services Department, Clwyd County Council
Mike McCarron	Social Work Department, Strathclyde Regional Council (representing the Convention of Scottish Local Authorities)
Denise Platt	Association of Metropolitan Authorities
Cynthia Spicer	Social Services Department, Kent County Council (representing the Association of County Councils)
Roy Taylor	Director of Social Services, Kingston-upon-Thames Borough Council (representing the Association of Directors of Social Services)
Pauline Thompson	Disablement Income Group
Representatives of	Department of Health
	DHSS, Northern Ireland
	The Scottish Office
	Welsh Office
	Department of Social Security

(DoH/Scottish Office/Welsh Office/Northern Ireland Office, 1996, p 15)

impairments under the age of 65). This would rule out people aged 65 and over and anybody without a physical impairment, although the government was particularly keen to consult on whether or not people under 65 with learning difficulties should be eligible for direct payments if willing and able to manage them (DoH/Scottish Office/Welsh Office/Northern Ireland Office, 1996, pp 4-5):

- Adults who have physical impairments (including people with sensory impairments), who are under the age of 65 and are able and willing to manage direct payments (with help if necessary). This does not exclude people with both a physical impairment and another condition (such as learning disability). Those aged 65 or over who began to receive direct payments before age 65 could continue to do so after that age.
- All disabled adults under the age of 65 who are able and willing to manage direct payments (with help if necessary). Those aged 65 or over who began to receive direct payments before age 65 could continue to do so after that age.
- All adults under the age of 65 who are able and willing to manage direct payments (with help if necessary). Those aged 65 or over who began to receive direct payments before age 65 could continue to do so after that age.
- All adults with physical impairments (including people with sensory impairments) who are able and willing to manage direct payments (with

Box 18: Restricting direct payments

The Bill gives the appropriate Secretary of State the power to specify in regulations which groups of people will be eligible to receive direct payments. Because this is a new departure, in order to give local authorities the best opportunity to implement direct payments effectively, the Government proposes to use this power to limit eligibility to a relatively small group in the first instance. Using regulations to specify who may receive the payments will make it possible for eligibility to be extended in the light of experience without the need for further primary legislation.

It is likely that direct payments will be popular and many people may wish to receive them. But this is a new and untested development. Experience with Independent Living Funds and with payment schemes operated by voluntary organisations will be useful, but direct payments have not previously been part of mainstream community care provision. Restricting the size of the eligible group will allow local authorities to test out direct payments on a limited scale, identifying and addressing any problems before the Government considers whether eligibility should be extended to others who are able and willing to manage direct payments. The Government thinks that this approach will give direct payments the greatest chance of being implemented successfully. (DoH/Scottish Office/Welsh Office/Northern Ireland Office, 1996, pp 3-4)

help if necessary), with no age limit. This does not exclude people who have both a physical impairment and another condition (such as learning disability).

- All disabled adults who are able and willing to manage direct payments (with help if necessary), with no age limit.
- All adults who are able and willing to manage direct payments (with help if necessary), with no age limit.

Another key issue in the consultation paper was a restriction on using direct payments to employ partners or close relatives (see Chapters Six, Eight and Nine for further discussion). This was justified by a desire to prevent existing informal care arrangements from becoming too formalised, to prevent the risk of exploitation and to prevent family members from feeling under pressure to give up their jobs and become full-time carers. However, a more cynical (and possibly more accurate) interpretation might be that it would prove too expensive to pay family carers for work which they had previously been expected to carry out free of charge as a result of their family obligations.

> The reason for the proposed restriction is to avoid creating pressure for informal care arrangements to be put on a formal, contractual basis. The relationships which people have with their informal carers (family or friends) is very different from their relationships with their employees. Direct payments will be an alternative to services which people would otherwise receive from the local authority – not to replace existing support networks within families and

> communities. If there were no restriction, there is a danger that direct payments recipients might come under pressure to employ family members when that would not be their choice. Conversely, parents or spouses who do not wish to give up their employment might find it difficult to resist pressure to give up their job and take on full-time care if there would be no loss of income. (DoH/Scottish Office/Welsh Office/Northern Ireland Office, 1996, p 8)

As a result of the government's determination to reserve the power to restrict eligibility to direct payments, the 1996 Community Care (Direct Payments) Act was relatively concise, with the bulk of detail provided through accompanying regulations (Statutory Instrument (SI) 1997/734) and subsequent policy and practice guidance (see Chapter Four). As the government had already indicated in the 1996 consultation paper, this would mean that the user groups eligible for direct payments could be expanded at a later stage if the experiment proved successful without the need for further legislation. As a result, the Act itself simply authorised local authorities to make payments directly to disabled people (see Box 19), with the bulk of the reforms to be set out in much greater detail by the Secretary of State. Under SI 1997/734, direct payments were to come into force in England and Wales on 1 April 1997, but were to exclude people 65 or over (unless payments started before the person's 65th birthday). Payments were not to be used for more than four weeks' residential care in any period of 12 months and could not be used to employ certain types of relatives and household members (see Chapter Four). Further SI and Statutory Rules (SRs) introduced direct payments to other parts of the country, including Scotland, Northern Ireland and the Isles of Scilly (SI 1996/1923 [NI 19]; SI 1997/693 [S 53]; SI 1997/759; SR 1997/131 and 133 [C6]). Thanks to ongoing lobbying by organisations of disabled people, the government's original intention to exclude people with learning difficulties from direct payments was defeated and direct payments were to be available to all adult user groups under the age of 65 (Care Plan, 1996a; Collins, 1996).

Box 19: The 1996 Community Care (Direct Payments) Act

Be it enacted by the Queen's most Excellent Majesty, by and with the advice and consent of the Lords Spiritual and Temporal, and Commons, in this present Parliament assembled, and by the authority of the same, as follows:

Where an authority have decided ... that the needs of a person call for the provision of any community care services ... the authority may, if the person consents, make to him, in respect of his securing the provision of any of the services for which they have decided his needs call, a payment of such amount as ... they think fit.

SUMMARY

As more and more groups of disabled people and local authorities began to experiment with various forms of payment schemes, pressure mounted in parliament to amend the NHS and Community Care Bill in order to support and promote the concept of direct payments. Despite significant campaigning by groups of disabled people and by a number of influential supporters, direct payments were declared illegal and draft legislation defeated. As the debate over direct payments raged, supporters emphasised the choice and control that payments could bring, while opponents voiced concerns that direct payments would be too complex and expensive to administer, creating a level of demand that could not be met. Although opposition was eventually overcome, direct payments were initially limited to particular user groups and restrictions were placed on the type of people that could be employed. Despite this, the legalisation of direct payments must be seen as a major victory for disabled people, who developed their own payments schemes in the 1980s and 1990s, carried out a sustained lobbying campaign, commissioned their own extremely influential research and participated in debates about how direct payments would operate. Although progress was slow, disabled campaigners and their allies were ultimately successful in prompting a major government re-think on the issue of direct payments and in furthering the goals of the Independent Living Movement.

Note

[1] The authors have been unable to obtain a copy of the original survey (Browne, 1990) from the author of the study, RADAR, or the British library, and have consequently had to rely on secondary literature.

FOUR

From indirect to direct payments II: guidance and extension

This chapter examines the policy and practice guidance that accompanied the introduction of direct payments and the subsequent extension of direct payments to new user groups. Under the 2001 Health and Social Care Act, the Secretary of State for Health can now issue regulations requiring local authorities to make direct payments to an individual who fulfils the requirements of the scheme and agrees to be part of it (see page 46).

Policy and practice guidance

After the passage of the 1996 Community Care (Direct Payments) Act, official policy and practice guidance was issued in May 1997 (DoH, 1997a; see Department of Health, Social Services and Public Safety, 1997; National Assembly for Wales, 1997; Scottish Office, 1997 for further details of direct payments in Scotland, Wales and Northern Ireland). This guidance was later revised and improved (see page 42 and DoH, 2000a).

Whereas the 1997 policy guidance set out *what* local authorities should do if they chose to exercise their new power to make direct payments, the practice guidance advised on *how* authorities might implement the Act. From the very beginning, the *policy guidance* emphasised that the government's aim was to enhance the independence of service users by giving them control over the way that community care services are delivered. To maximise this independence, local authorities should work in partnership with disabled people and leave as much choice as possible in the hands of the service user, while at the same time ensuring that the individual's needs are being met and that public money is being used appropriately and cost-effectively. Although authorities now have the *power* to make direct payments, they do not have a *duty* to do so and retain discretion over:

- whether or not to implement direct payments;
- for which services (if any) payments are available;
- whether to arrange some services for users as well as making payments;
- whether or not to offer someone a direct payment;
- how much flexibility individual recipients have over the way the money is spent;
- how much of a payment to make and what it is supposed to cover.

Whatever the authority decides to do, it should not treat direct payment recipients any more, or less, favourably than people receiving services and should continue to develop other ways of making services more responsive.

Since payments are only to be made by local authority social services departments in lieu of community care services, they are only to be given to people assessed as needing community care services. Although they cannot be used to make payments to any other body (for example, a health or housing authority), the guidance anticipates that there might be some situations in which a health authority contributes funds to a package of social care (see Chapters Seven and Eight for further discussion). In such cases it would be acceptable to use these funds to contribute to a direct payments package, providing that the payments are given by the social services department for social care services. Although direct payments can be used for all community care services, this excludes permanent residential care (including a total of more than four weeks' respite care in any 12-month period) and services provided directly by the local authority. Since direct payments are an alternative to community care services, authorities offering payments will need to do so within their existing budgets (see Chapter Eight for a further discussion of financial issues).

The original legislation prevents payments to people under 18 or to adults wishing to purchase services for people aged under 18. Although users may ask carers, or other third parties, to help them manage direct payments, the user must remain in control of the payment and is accountable for the way the money is used. Initially, direct payments were to be made available only to disabled people under 65 (including people with physical impairments, learning difficulties, mental health problems and HIV/AIDS), although people receiving such payments before the age of 65 could carry on receiving them after that age. However, this was to be reviewed after the Act had been in force for one year. In addition, direct payments could not be offered to certain people in the mental health or criminal justice system, including:

- patients detained under mental health legislation who are on leave of absence from hospital;
- conditionally discharged detained patients subject to Home Office restrictions;
- patients subject to guardianship under mental health legislation;
- people under supervised discharge under the 1995 Mental Health (Patients in the Community) Act;
- people receiving aftercare;
- offenders serving a probation or community order subject to an additional requirement to undergo treatment for a mental health condition or for drug/alcohol dependency;
- offenders released on licence subject to an additional requirement to undergo treatment for a mental health condition or for drug/alcohol dependency;
- people subject to equivalent Scottish mental health/criminal justice legislation.

Other key features of the guidance are summarised below:

1. Community care plans should include input from direct payment users and local authorities should consult interested parties before considering how to implement the Act locally. Information should be readily available and accessible (see Chapter Eight for a further discussion), and the views of users and carers should be taken into account as part of the monitoring and reviewing of direct payment schemes.

2. In situations where an authority is considering offering a direct payment, assessments should include a consideration of the individual's capacity to manage direct payments and time for the service user to consider the implications of receiving direct payments. To aid this process, authorities should raise the possibility of direct payments at an early stage, allow the user as much time as possible to think about this option and provide as much information as possible about the implications of receiving direct payments. Direct payments should only be offered to people who the authority considers are able to manage them (alone or with assistance). Although authorities may refuse payments to anyone who they feel is unable to manage them, they should take this decision on an individual basis and should avoid blanket assumptions that whole groups of people are unable to manage payments. While people may receive assistance with managing the money, they are accountable for the way it is spent, must retain ultimate control over the payment and should be able to overrule any decision made on their behalf by an agent (see Chapter Six for a further discussion of issues of capacity and ability to manage direct payments). Although there is no restriction on who may help a user manage their money, the authority should satisfy itself that adequate help is available and be aware of possible conflicts of interest.

3. Direct payments may only be made to people who consent to receive them, and local authorities should satisfy themselves that service users understand the financial and legal responsibilities they are undertaking. In particular, authorities must explain what is involved in receiving payments as fully as possible and draw people's attention to the legal responsibilities that direct payments will bring, making it clear that services can be provided in a normal way if someone decides against direct payments. Authorities should also discuss how users will secure the services they have been assessed as needing and how their direct payments should be used.

4. Payments may not be used to purchase services from a partner or a close relative living in the same household. In addition, services cannot be purchased from a close relative living elsewhere or from someone else living in the same household, although authorities may make an exception to this rule if this is the only appropriate way of securing the relevant services. For the purposes of the Act, a close relative is defined as a parent, parent-in-law, aunt, uncle, grandparent, son, daughter, son-in-law, daughter-in-law, step son or

daughter, brother, sister or the spouse or partners of any of the above. This restriction is not meant to prevent disabled people from employing live-in PAs, but should prevent recipients employing people with whom they have a personal, rather than a contractual, relationship (see Chapters Six, Eight and Nine for further discussion).

5. Crucially, local authorities should only make a direct payment if this will be at least as cost-effective as the services that would otherwise be arranged. In making this decision, authorities should consider the full cost of a direct payment and the cost of the equivalent services (including administrative costs and overheads). While an authority may make payments at a greater cost than the cost of directly provided services, it may only do so if this is as cost-effective as arranging services (that is, if the cost if justified by the greater effectiveness arising from enabling the person to manage their own services and live independently).

6. In deciding how much of a payment to make, authorities must ensure that their payments enable recipients legally to secure a service of a sufficient standard to meet the needs for which the payment is made. Recipients can use their own resources to purchase additional or better services, and can be asked to make a financial contribution to the cost of their care. For charging purposes, authorities should treat people receiving direct payments as they would treat anyone else under their charging policy (see Chapters Seven and Eight for further discussion of financial and cost-efficiency issues).

7. Once direct payments have begun, authorities must be satisfied that users' assessed needs are being met and that the money is being spent appropriately. Although authorities may set conditions to ensure the proper use of public funds, they cannot set unnecessary conditions and should not limit the direct payment recipient to certain providers. At the same time, authorities will need to review care packages on a regular basis and monitor the way in which payments are being used to ensure that assessed needs are being met and that public funds are being used appropriately (see Chapter Eight for further discussion of financial and accountability issues). Although authorities should discuss the contingency plans that users will make, they will be responsible for arranging services if care arrangements break down. If an authority is not satisfied that direct payments have been used to secure the services to which the payments relate, it can require some, or all, of the money to be repaid. However, this power should not be used to penalise genuine mistakes and should be discussed with users before they begin receiving payments. Either the authority or the user may decide to discontinue direct payments at any time, although authorities should set a minimum period of notice (unless there are exceptional circumstances) and explain the circumstances in which payments might be stopped in advance. If discontinuation is necessary and the user also receives ILF payments, the authority should also contact the ILF. If service users are dissatisfied with

> the authority at any stage, they should have the same access to the social services complaints system as users of directly provided services.

Drawing on the experience of current independent living schemes, the *practice guidance* emphasises that service users are well placed to judge how best to use direct payments and have a vested interest in using their payments properly on necessary services. The guidance acknowledges that direct payments can be complex, but states that "the aim should be to set up simple but effective systems, which contain safeguards but are not unnecessarily bureaucratic or time-consuming" (DoH, 1997a, p 26). Since direct payments are intended to enhance control, this process should begin at the very start through consultations with people with different types of impairment, people from different ethnic backgrounds and people of different ages. In cases where direct payments may be offered, it may be helpful for authorities to put people in touch with a support group or a local centre for independent living before an assessment of need takes place (see also Chapter Eight). During the assessment itself, the more involved the user becomes in decisions about direct payments, the greater the chance of a successful care package. To help the person make an informed decision, it may be useful to give them a Department of Health information booklet (1998b).

When deciding how direct payments are to be used, authorities may wish to seek legal advice and should help service users obtain information about local services which they might purchase. However, authorities should not be constrained by existing services and should explore innovative and creative ways of meeting a user's needs. Although authorities can decide whether or not to allow direct payments to be used for purchasing equipment, this may not be a cost-effective option in the case of specialist equipment (which may require considerable expertise to ensure that the equipment is safe and appropriate). Authorities should also clarify the ownership of equipment, and responsibilities for ongoing care and maintenance. Once a package of care has been agreed, care plans should set out what has been decided, making clear what the money may be spent on, how much flexibility the user has and the information which the user will have to provide for audit purposes (see Box 20 for a checklist). In deciding the amount of a direct payment, authorities will need to discuss the arrangements which users are intending to make and associated costs such as National Insurance, sick pay, maternity pay, liability insurance and VAT (see Chapter Eight for further discussion). Authorities can decide how to make payments and whether to do so in arrears or in advance, but may also need to set up procedures for making additional payments in emergencies.

In particular, the practice guidance emphasises the importance of adequate support mechanisms. This might include access to someone with employment expertise, a payroll service, lists of local agencies, assistance with drafting advertisements, job descriptions and contracts, rooms for interviewing, training, advocacy or written materials (see Chapters Eight and Nine). Above all, however, direct payment recipients may benefit from peer support:

> Experience with independent living projects suggests that direct payments will work best where people who receive the payments have access to support as they manage the money, particularly in the early stages. The Government encourages local authorities to arrange for people to whom they make direct payments to have access to such support. This might be by providing a service directly, in partnership with a local voluntary organisation, or by some other means.... The experience of users on existing independent living schemes is that they find it easier to seek advice from someone who is independent of the local authority.... People who have experience of managing direct payments themselves are well placed to advise and help others as they begin to receive direct payments. In many areas, people who are managing their own care meet regularly to support one another and to discuss any difficulties which have arisen. This can be an effective way of sharing experience. (DoH, 1997a, pp 39-40)

In monitoring and reviewing direct payment packages, authorities should ask themselves how they would know if someone was experiencing difficulties managing their payments. For audit purposes, it will have to be possible to identify direct payments money separately from any other money used for similar purposes (for example, ILF payments). Despite this, audit arrangements should be as simple and easy to understand as possible, avoiding needless intrusion (see Chapter Eight). Although difficulties can be minimised by good practice when considering, making and monitoring direct payments, users may wish to have a named contact in case of emergency. If difficulties do arise, the social services department may wish to ask itself the following:

- Have the person's needs changed?
- Is the amount of money sufficient to enable the person to secure the relevant services?
- Is the person still able to manage direct payments?
- Does the person wish to continue receiving direct payments?
- Has all the money been spent on the services for which it was intended?
- Have the services for which the user has paid been received?
- Has the money been spent wisely?

To support the implementation of direct payments, the policy and practice guidance was followed by speaking notes/overhead templates for a presentation on direct payments, a guide to receiving direct payments and two promotional videos (DoH, 1997b, 1998b, 1998c, 1999). Although the presentation materials tended to summarise the more detailed policy and practice guidance, they also included a number of additional statements of the government's intent. Thus, it was emphasised from the beginning that direct payments are based on three central principles (DoH, 1997b, para 2):

- Direct payments are about increasing user independence.
- Direct payments are about increasing user choice.

- Direct payments work best when they are introduced as a partnership between the local authority and the direct payment recipient.

Box 20: Care plan for direct payments – checklist

- What are the person's needs as identified in the assessment?
- To which of these needs do the direct payments relate?
- How will the person secure the appropriate services?
- What variations to the way in which the direct payments are used does the authority expect to be asked in advance to approve?
- What support (if any) does the user need to manage their direct payments?
- How will this support be made available to the person?
- What arrangements has the person made to cover emergencies?
- How much money does the authority consider necessary to secure the appropriate services?
- How much of this total will the authority contribute in direct payments, and how much is the person expected to contribute?
- How often and in what form will payments be made?
- What arrangements does the authority propose for monitoring? What information should the person provide? What access will be required to the person's home?
- What information does the authority require for audit purposes and when?
- What, if any, other conditions are attached to the direct payment?
- When will the next review take place?
- What should the person do if he or she wants to stop receiving direct payments?
- In what circumstances will the authority consider discontinuing payments?
- How will the authority and user handle any temporary gap in direct payments being made?
- How much notice will be given if the authority discontinues?
- How will any outstanding commitments be handled if direct payments are discontinued?
- In what circumstances would direct payments be withdrawn with no notice?
- In what circumstances would the authority seek repayment?

(DoH, 1997a, p 49)

Building on previous work, the presentation materials summarised the key features of developing partnerships with users and carers (see Box 21). At the same time, the presentation pack also sought to explain the emphasis of the 1997 guidance on users being willing and able to manage their own payments, suggesting that direct payments were designed to enhance independence, not to transfer dependence from a local authority to dependence on a third party.

In the Department of Health's (1998b) *Guide to receiving direct payments* the government provided information about the nature of direct payments legislation and how to purchase personal assistance. To make the guide as accessible as possible, it was written in large print and was also available in Braille, in audio tape format and in a range of community languages. Based on a

Box 21: Partnership working

Working in partnership with users and carers means:

- Listening to what they want and not making assumptions about their wishes.
- Respecting their opinions and taking account of what they say.
- Involving them in decisions both individually at a personal level and collectively in planning, commissioning, delivering and monitoring services.
- Including them in the difficult decisions, when there are hard choices to be made, as well as in the simple or easy decisions.
- Providing them with full information and making sure they know what options and choices are open to them.
- Supporting them in the choices they make.

(DoH, 1997b, para 6)

question and answer format, the guide explains how to get direct payments, how to become an employer, how to contract with someone who is self-employed and how to contract with an agency, providing readers with contacts for further information and setting out a range of useful publications. This includes details of how to obtain further information about the responsibilities involved in becoming an employer (see Box 22).

In the first of the promotional videos, *Independence pays*, the government emphasises the choice and control inherent in direct payments (see Box 23), interviewing staff and service users at the Kingston-upon-Thames Independent Living Scheme (DoH, 1998c). This project was first established in the late 1980s when the social services department was approached by a number of

Box 22: Becoming an employer

Being an employer involves new responsibilities and direct payment recipients should consider a range of issues:

- Providing a written statement of employment particulars
- Protecting against unfair dismissal
- Giving periods of notice
- Deducting tax
- National Insurance contributions
- Statutory sick pay
- Maternity pay
- Redundancy pay
- Equal opportunities
- The right to belong to a trades union
- Employers' Liability Insurance
- Health and safety issues.

(DoH, 1998b, Appendix A)

Box 23: Choice and control

"I feel that it [the direct payments scheme] has enabled me to lead a fairly independent life."

"It's given me more control. I can ask people to come in when I want them."

"It's meant me having control over my life."

"It's made the world of difference."

"It's changed the way I feel about myself. It's given me status, friends, work."

(DoH, 1998c)

disabled people with a view to making payments instead of providing services. From the beginning, the scheme sought to combine choice and control with the need for public accountability. As the scheme progressed, the authority found that direct payments spread primarily through word of mouth as people with positive experiences of direct payments shared information with friends. Although receiving direct payments brings added responsibilities, local disabled people responded by establishing a peer support group, with advice being available from a social services worker. Although the scheme was not felt to lead to large reductions in expenditure, it was perceived as being more cost-effective than traditional services since the disabled people concerned were able to be more creative and innovative than the social services department in deciding how to use their payments. Presided over by Roy Taylor, Director of Community Services in Kingston-upon-Thames and a chair of the ADSS Disabilities Committee, the Kingston scheme has attracted more publicity than most direct payment projects (see, for example, Macfarlane, 1990 or Webb, 1996).

In a second video designed for the Deaf community, the government made information available to disabled people with a narrator using sign language (with subtitles and a voiceover) (DoH, 1999). A key message was that direct payments could be a flexible and practical option for people with sensory impairments, enabling Deaf people to employ PAs who sign or people with visual impairments to access community resources. In one case study authority (Barnet), direct payments were being used to purchase specialist equipment such as minicoms or textphones. Overall, the narrator concluded that "direct payments are about more than just enabling you to get the kind of support you need, they are about allowing you to make your own decisions and live the way you want to" (DoH, 1999).

The extension of direct payments

When direct payments were implemented in April 1997, policy and practice guidance emphasised that the reforms would be reviewed after one year of operation with a view to reconsidering the user groups eligible for direct payments (DoH, 1997a). Since the original 1996 Act and 1997 guidance, three main developments have taken place:

- the extension of direct payments to older people;
- revised policy and practice guidance;
- the extension of direct payments to carers, people with parental responsibility for disabled children and disabled young people.

On 1 February 2000, new regulations removed the age limit that had initially applied to direct payments, enabling people aged 65 and over to benefit from such payments in authorities that decided to take advantage of the new powers available to them (Age Concern, 2000; SI 2000/11). Although these regulations only applied to England at the time, similar changes have since taken place in Wales, Scotland and Northern Ireland (SI 2000/183; SI 2000/1868 (W127); SR 2000/114). Since older people are such a large and significant user group, this move was likely to have considerable implications for the future of direct payments and opinion is currently divided as to how popular this measure will prove among older people (see Chapter Six for further details).

In 1999/2000, the Department of Health issued revised policy and practice guidance to take account of the relatively slow progress to date in implementing direct payments and the recent extension of the scheme to older people (DoH, 2000a). Although the guidance was often very similar to its predecessor (and often repeated sections of the original guidance verbatim), there were a number of crucial changes which seemed to indicate the government's intention to increase the availability of direct payments and to ensure that particular groups of service users were not excluded. As a result, the guidance emphasises from the beginning that direct payments have a very broad potential, improving quality of life, promoting independence, aiding social inclusion and encompassing areas such as rehabilitation, education, leisure and employment. The government is clear that it "wants to see more extensive use made of direct payments" (DoH, 2000a, p 3) and that authorities will need to consider how to include people with different types of impairment, people from different ethnic backgrounds and people of different ages. When deciding whether or not to offer direct payments to an individual, authorities should not "fetter their discretion" (that is, they should consider each case on its merits, even where the authority is not currently offering direct payments and treat all adult client groups equitably) (DoH, 2000a, p 4). Although direct payments can still only be offered if they are at least as cost-effective as direct services, there is a recognition that any consideration of cost-effectiveness should consider long-term best value. Thus, the guidance is clear that:

> A preventive strategy may necessitate a slightly higher investment to achieve long-term benefits and savings. Provision of direct payments that allow a person to remain in their own home may represent long-term savings if that person does not require hospital or residential care. There may be savings both to the local authority and health authority. (DoH, 2000a, p 8)

In the practice guidance, there is particular emphasis on consulting older people (only recently enabled to receive direct payments) and groups such as people with sensory impairments or learning difficulties that may not be fully encompassed by many existing schemes. There is also even greater emphasis on the importance of adequate support than in the original 1997 guidance and a recognition that support should include information, advice, peer support and training as a minimum starting point. This is particularly the case with regard to people with learning difficulties, who may have little real knowledge about their current services and who will require accessible information about the care they already receive before making choices about future options.

At the same time as it issued revised guidance, the government also indicated its intention to introduce legislation to extend direct payments to a range of user groups and their carers originally excluded from the 1996 Act. In 1999, the Carers and Disabled Children Bill was introduced to Parliament and, on 20 July 2000, received royal assent (see Box 24). Under the Act, local authorities are empowered to make direct payments to three new groups of people (DoH, 2000c):

- carers (including 16- and 17-year-old carers) for services that meet their assessed needs;
- people with parental responsibility for disabled children for services to the family;
- 16- and 17-year-old disabled children for services that meet their own assessed needs.

As with the original 1996 Act, these changes were justified by the Department of Health on the grounds that they will lead to more flexible and responsive services:

> [Previous work with carers] was aimed at empowering carers to make more choices for themselves and to have more control over their lives. To that end, the Act extends direct payments legislation to carers to meet their own assessed needs. The extension of direct payments to 16 and 17 year old carers is designed to offer them additional flexibility in meeting their developmental needs. The responsibilities of persons with parental responsibility for disabled children are sometimes made more arduous by the difficulty of accessing mainstream services, for example child care, including after school clubs and leisure activities. Where these carers do not think services are sufficiently tailored to the needs of their family direct payments offer more choice in the ways services are delivered. The extension of direct payments to 16- and 17-year-old disabled

> children may be particularly helpful where those children are intending to leave home or residential care to go into further or higher education. (DoH, 2000c, paras 11 and 12)

After the Carers and Disabled Children Bill became an Act of Parliament, it was accompanied by a raft of policy and practice guidance (DoH, 2001a, b, c, d). Under the Act and guidance, authorities may make direct payments to:

- *Carers aged 16 and over*: "Direct payments will allow carers to purchase the services they are assessed as needing *as carers* to support them in their caring role and to maintain their own health and well being" (DoH, 2001b, p 12; emphasis in the original). The carer cannot receive payments to purchase services for the person they care for, and must remain in control of arrangements and accountable for the way in which the payment is used. Although direct payments are unlikely to be the best option for 16- and 17-year-old carers, it is possible to make such payments where the council supports the young person's decision to undertake a substantial caring role. In carrying out carers' assessments, practitioners are prompted to consider the appropriateness of direct payments (DoH, 2001d).
- *People with parental responsibility for disabled children*: Direct payments may be made to the parents of disabled children where the local council is satisfied that "the parent is a person who will make arrangements that are designed to safeguard and promote the welfare of the child" (DoH, 2001b, p 15). Payments may be used to purchase services to meet the assessed needs of the disabled child or to provide short-terms breaks which meet the needs of both parent and child. Councils have a duty to carry out checks under the 1999 Protection of Children Act via the Criminal Records Bureau when asked to do so by a parent wishing to use direct payments to employ an individual to care for their child (DoH, 2001a, b).
- *Young disabled people*: "The Carers and Disabled Children Act gives local councils ... the power to offer direct payments to 16 and 17 year old disabled people to enable them to arrange the provision of services that meet their assessed needs under the Children Act 1989 rather than rely on direct service provision from the local council" (DoH, 2001c, p 3). Where a disabled young person and their parents are in disagreement, the local authority should give preference to the young person's views (provided that the young person has sufficient understanding to make informed decisions). Where requested, the council should carry out checks on potential employees in the same way as for the parents of disabled children (as discussed above).

Despite these changes, the principles set out in the 2000 policy and practice guidance (DoH, 2000a) remain substantially unchanged with regard to issues such as charging, consent and ability to manage a direct payment.

Box 24: The 2000 Carers and Disabled Children Act

House of Commons	Date
Introduction	15 December 1999
Second Reading	4 February 2000
Committee	8 March 2000
	15 March 2000
Report and Third Reading	5 May 2000

House of Lords	Date
Introduction	9 May 2000
Second Reading	23 June 2000
Order of Commitment discharged	14 July 2000
Third Reading	20 July 2000

Source: DoH (2000c)

While the extension of direct payments has been broadly welcomed by many commentators, a number of concerns have been raised. To begin with, disability organisations, such as NCIL (2000a), have suggested that there is scope for conflict between users and carers, arguing that extending direct payments to other groups should not undermine the basic goal of increasing users' independence. Expanding direct payments will also raise the need for additional support services, and existing monitoring processes may need to be simplified for young people and carers. There is also anxiety concerning the contradiction between the current trend towards emphasising the value of carers' contribution on the one hand, and the decision to charge carers (and other recipients) for their direct payments on the other hand (NCIL, 2000a). At the same time, there also seem to be anomalies in the extended and revised direct payments scheme that will require further attention:

- Although the parents of children with profound learning difficulties may be able to receive direct payments, this will cease once the child becomes 18 in cases where the individual is not considered willing and able to manage their own payments. Although the government has previously indicated that it sees little point in transferring dependence on a local authority to dependence on a third party, there must surely be a case for allowing people with profound learning difficulties to benefit from the flexibility of direct payments. One option might be for payments to be administered on the person's behalf by a group of people chosen by, or significant to, the user (such as family members, friends, community figures and social care staff). (This issue is discussed in more detail in Chapter Six.)
- Despite more numerous references to people with learning difficulties and older people in the 2000 guidance, it is clear that the current system for making and monitoring direct payments is based primarily on the needs of people with physical impairments. Although the experience of different

user groups is discussed in greater detail in Chapter Six, key obstacles include the emphasis on being willing and able to manage direct payments, and the complexity of some of the monitoring processes established by local authorities to ensure public accountability.
- In deciding whether or not direct payments represent a cost-effective option, local authorities can consider long-term issues such as whether or not direct payments are likely to prevent a future hospital or residential care admission. This is a much wider definition of cost-efficiency than in the 1997 guidance and includes not only social services expenditure, but also possible savings to outside agencies such as the NHS. If direct payments are to be used to make long-term savings in both health and social care, is there a case for extending the scope of direct payments beyond social services provision? (For further details see Chapter Eight.)

At the time of writing, Parliament has recently passed the 2001 Health and Social Care Act. Under Section 57 of the Act, it will be possible to make regulations that may require local authorities to make direct payments to a service user who fulfils certain criteria and consents to receiving such payments (DoH, 2001e, para 274). While the exact nature of the intentions behind the Act is not currently clear, this would seem to indicate a commitment by central government to increase the number of people receiving direct payments, and a move from a discretionary to a mandatory system:

> Section 57 deals with direct payments in respect of adults. Under the current system local authorities are permitted but not required to offer direct payments to people who meet the eligibility criteria. Subsection (1) allows regulations to be made to make provision for and in connection with requiring or authorising a local authority to make direct payments to an individual who fulfils the requirements of the scheme and agrees to be part of it.

Further change is also likely in Scotland, where the Deputy Minister for Health and Community Care, Malcolm Chisholm, has announced that £530,000 is to be allocated over a two-year period to a new development project led by a consortium of voluntary organisations and user-led agencies. The project aims to:

- set up/develop existing user-led support groups;
- provide training, guidance and build confidence at local levels;
- coordinate and provide feedback to the Scottish Executive;
- increase awareness of direct payments at local and national levels;
- establish mechanisms for information sharing (Scottish Executive, 2001).

In addition to the development project, Chisholm has hinted at even greater changes to come:

> Direct payments are the future for disabled people. We want to raise awareness of these schemes and ensure they become more accessible throughout Scotland. As part of that process, the Scottish Executive is preparing to consult with clients, families and carers, and statutory and voluntary agencies on how we can make sure they are available to all disabled people who want them.... While not all disabled people will want to receive direct payments, we believe that the choice should be theirs. (Scottish Executive, 2001)

Such an approach has also received support from the Scottish Executive's Care Development Group, whose report on free personal care for older people in residential/nursing homes recommended that direct payments should be available to "all those who want them" (Care Development Group, 2001, p 63). Other key measures being debated and/or implemented in Scotland include:

- The relaxation of the ban of using direct payments to purchase local authority services and on employing close relatives living in a different household.
- The extension of direct payments to guardians and attorneys for people unable to manage their own payments (Scottish Executive 2000, 2001).

SUMMARY

Since 1996, the Community Care (Direct Payments) Act has been followed by detailed policy and practice guidance which defines the responsibilities of local authorities and clarifies how direct payments are to operate. This has been accompanied by a range of publicity material designed to promote the reforms. Although payments were initially restricted to people between the ages of 18 and 65, they have since been extended to a range of new user groups, with revised guidance. At the time of writing, there is every indication that the current government is firmly committed to the concept of direct payments and intends to act in order to make such payments mandatory rather than simply discretionary. Although subsequent chapters highlight the slow progress of direct payments and the difficulties experienced by particular user groups, it is possible that direct payments will become an increasingly significant feature of social services provision in the future.

FIVE

The progress of direct payments

Although the passage of the 1996 Community Care (Direct Payments) Act was a major victory for disabled campaigners, the legislation was permissive rather than mandatory (see Chapters Three and Four). Amid considerable concerns about the cost implications of the new scheme, it was perhaps inevitable that while some authorities would choose to implement direct payments almost immediately, others would be more cautious and possibly even hostile to the 1996 Act. This has resulted in a situation where the rate of implementation has been extremely uneven, creating something of a postcode lottery. Although more and more authorities are starting to introduce direct payment schemes, and although the 2001 Health and Social Care Act empowers the Secretary of State to issue regulations requiring authorities to make direct payments, major barriers still remain. Against this background, this chapter reviews the pace of implementation, highlighting key obstacles to progress. For comparative purposes, reference will also be made to the European Independent Living Movement and to the different direct payment schemes that have been developed in a number of countries.

Early days

As noted in Chapter Three, research carried out by the PSI two years prior to the Community Care (Direct Payments) Act suggested that many authorities were already making payments to service users and that many more would do so if legislation permitted (see Tables 1 and 2).

Despite this, there were considerable regional variations, with availability gradually moving from the south to the north and the west of Britain. While 80% of respondents in London were making payments, this was true of only 17% of respondents in the North West, 25% in Wales, 33% in the South West and 40% in the West Midlands (see Table 3). The researchers were also at pains to stress that many local authorities were only making payments to a small

Table 1: Availability of direct/indirect payments (1994)

	Number of authorities	%
Authorities making direct payments	4	5
Authorities making indirect payments	44	54
Do not make payments	34	41
Totals (response rate = 64%)	**82**	**100**

Source: Zarb and Nadash (1994, p 26)

Table 2: Local authorities who would make payments if legislation permitted

	Number of authorities	%
Authorities who would make direct payments	76	93
Authorities who would make indirect payments	3	4
Undecided	3	4
Totals (response rate = 64%)	**82**	**101**

Source: Zarb and Nadash (1994, p 26)

Table 3: Regional variations

Region	Proportion of participating authorities making payments (%)
Greater London	80
South	78
South East	50
South West	33
East Anglia	50
West Midlands	40
East Midlands	50
North West	17
North East	27
Scotland	64
Wales	25

Source: Zarb and Nadash (1994, p 27)

number of people (Zarb and Nadash, 1994, p 27). Overall, the only exception to the concentration of payment schemes in the south was Scotland, where such payments had been legal for some time (see page 55).

After the legalisation of direct payments under the 1996 Act, progress in England and Wales has not been as rapid as Zarb and Nadash's (1994) initial research might have suggested. In 1997, the PSI and NCIL published preliminary findings from a research study into the implementation and management of direct payments (Zarb et al, 1997). Based on a survey of all UK local authorities and on more detailed consultations with 10 selected authorities, the research suggested that under 50% of local authorities were operating some form of payments scheme and that many were unsure whether to introduce such payments in the future (see Tables 4 and 5). Although London, the South West and Scotland had been relatively proactive, provision was very low in the north of England, Wales and Northern Ireland (see Table 6). For many local authorities, the main concerns over the implementation and management of direct payments were found to include:

- financial monitoring and review;
- ensuring that support purchased meets users' needs;
- assessing users' ability to manage payments and/or support arrangements;
- the provision of support and advice for users.

Table 4: Direct payment schemes (June-July 1997)

Current provision	Percentage of local authorities (*n*=185)
No payments	52
Third party payments	31
Other payment arrangements (for example, combination of direct/indirect payments or payments through trusts)	11
Direct payments	6

Source: Adapted from Zarb et al (1997, p 2)

Table 5: Plans to introduce direct payments

Plans to introduce direct payments (authorities without existing schemes)	Percentage of local authorities (*n*=97)
Planning to introduce payments	65
Don't know/undecided	33
Not planning to make payments	2

Source: Adapted from Zarb et al (1997, p 3)

Table 6: Regional variations (June-July 1997)

Region	Percentage of local authorities providing payments schemes
South West	85
Scotland	76
Greater London	70
East Midlands	62
South East	53
East Anglia	33
West Midlands	33
Yorkshire and Humberside	27
North	23
North West	23
Wales	10
Northern Ireland	0

Source: Adapted from Zarb et al (1997, p 4)

England and Wales

In autumn 1998, the Department of Health distributed a questionnaire among all English local authorities to monitor the implementation of the 1996 Act (Auld, 1999). Of 150 authorities, 135 (90%) returned the questionnaire. These responses suggested that 68 (51%) respondents were operating direct payment schemes and that direct payments were being made to 1,404 people, the vast majority of whom were people with physical impairments (see Chapter Six for further details). Of the 67 authorities not operating schemes, 59 (88%) indicated that they intended to set up schemes. Once again, there were significant regional differences, both in the number of authorities who had implemented direct payments and in the number of people receiving such payments (see Table 7).

In 1999, the Social Services Inspectorate (SSI) undertook a national programme of inspections to examine how councils promoted independent living arrangements for disabled people aged 18 to 65 (Fruin, 2000). Inspections took place in 10 councils, chosen to be broadly representative of all English local authorities (see Box 25). Overall, the inspectors were "disappointed at the limited progress made by most of the sampled councils in introducing direct payments". Only one council had as many as 20 users, further work was required to extend and publicise schemes and most councils needed to pay greater attention to promoting peer support, self-help groups and voluntary sector input (Fruin, 2000, p 3).

Table 7: Regional variations (autumn 1998)

Region	Number (%) authorities operating direct payments	Number of people receiving direct payments
Central	11 (44)	74
London	20 (67)	145
North	16 (36)	176
South	21 (60)	1,009
Total	**68 (51)**	**1,404**

Source: Auld (1999)

Box 25: Direct payments in 10 English authorities (1999)

Brighton and Hove had responded positively to the introduction of direct payments, establishing a pilot project in 1997 for eight service users. After an evaluation, proposals were being considered to develop the scheme for people with a care package of at least 10 hours, with a possible extension to people with HIV/AIDS and people with learning difficulties. Accessible information and guidance were available to users, but a support group of direct payment users had not yet been formed.

Calderdale did not have a direct payments scheme, but was seeking to set one up. It was proposed that this scheme would only initially be for people with physical impairments, although the inspectors noted that they had met some people with learning difficulties who wished to explore this option and recommended that the scheme should be available to both groups.

Enfield did not have a direct payments scheme, although three people were receiving payments negotiated individually prior to the 1996 Direct Payments Act. These people had no links with other service users and no specialised support. Proposals had been developed for a scheme for 12 people to be introduced in 2000, although there was no network of service users able to provide peer support or independent advocacy.

Herefordshire had introduced a pilot direct payments scheme, supported by Herefordshire Centre for Independent Living. Although the scheme was deemed to be successful, senior managers were concerned about its affordability and the future was uncertain.

Lincolnshire had established a direct payments pilot in 1997 for around 20 users and there was a firm commitment to extending the scheme. While direct payments were viewed positively by recipients, there was some confusion over levels of payments, the needs that the scheme could be used to meet and whether day care or leisure activities were included. Since different workers had adopted different interpretations, there was a degree of inequity and confusion among recipients. Other service users felt that the scheme was too complex and bureaucratic. Although comprehensive information was available, 36% of direct payment users surveyed by the inspectors did not know how to get more information and 50% did not know how to ask for changes to their service.

Middlesbrough had not been able to implement direct payments. Although proposals to establish pilot schemes had been developed and approved in 1997, the pilots had not materialised and the inspectors had little confidence that direct payments would be introduced.

Oxfordshire had made direct payments available in April 1998 and the scheme had 14 users, supported by an independent advice service. A key local concern was the difficulty of recruiting PAs.

Poole had established a pilot scheme and was in the process of making this part of mainstream services available to all user groups. There were seven people using the scheme with a further four being assessed. The scheme was supported by an independent living Coordinator and all (120) recipients of domiciliary care with physical or sensory impairments had been informed in writing about direct payments. The scheme was limited to a maximum of 63 hours personal care per week.

Stockport did not operate a direct payments scheme due to restrictions on management time, although research had been undertaken and a pilot was planned for April 2000.

Westminster had a small direct payments scheme with six recipients. Plans were underway to expand the scheme, extend it to people with learning difficulties and make support services available. (DoH/SSI, 1999a-1999j)

In summer 2000, the ADSS surveyed all 171 social services departments in England and Wales with a response rate of 100% (Jones, 2000). This study found that 80% of authorities had introduced direct payment schemes and that all bar one of the remaining 20% planned to follow suit (see Table 8). Despite this, strong regional variations remained, with direct payments most prominent in London and the South, and much less so in Wales. Around 3,500 people were receiving direct payments, although a number of authorities had excluded people with mental health problems and/or learning difficulties from their schemes (see Chapter Six for further details). The report concluded in upbeat fashion:

> The survey results ... indicated some regional variations in the availability of direct payments, but if the authorities currently not providing direct payments follow up on their plans *there should soon be almost total availability across England and Wales of direct payments*.... The task now is for social services to work with disabled people to increase the take-up of direct payments, and to make direct payments a mainstream opportunity, as one means of promoting independent living. (Jones, 2000; emphasis in the original)

Although the researchers cited above have not sought to explore in detail the concentration of direct payments in particular regions, it is clear that there are a number of individual authorities that heavily influence national overviews. In the case of the ADSS research (Jones, 2000), the authorities with the largest number of direct payment users were identified as Hampshire (400), Essex (239), Southampton (133), Sheffield (100) and North Yorkshire (98). While few commentators have attempted to explain the predominance of a small handful of authorities, it is interesting to note that some of the authorities with the most direct payment users correlate with areas with a well-established and/or active Independent Living Movement. This is particularly the case in Hampshire – the home of the first indirect payment scheme in Britain (see Chapter Three).

Table 8: Direct payments in England and Wales (2000)

Region	Number of authorities with direct payments	Percentage with direct payments	Number of people receiving direct payments
London	31	94	414
Central	27	93	808
South	32	76	1,740
North	32	70	571
Wales	14	66	79
Total	**136**	**80**	**3,612**

Source: Adapted from Jones (2000)

Scotland

In Scotland, direct payments have technically been legal since the 1968 Social Work (Scotland) Act. Under section 12 of the Act, authorities can make direct payments or payments in kind, but only in exceptional circumstances where a cash payment would be cheaper than other forms of assistance (see Box 26). This legislation was subsequently amended under the 1996 Community Care (Direct Payments) Act and new guidance introduced (Scottish Office, 1997).

Despite the different legislative framework operating in Scotland from 1968 to 1996, Zarb and Nadash (1994) found that only 64% of Scottish authorities were making payments (either direct or indirect) and that a few were not even aware that they were permitted to make payments under the 1968 Act. Due to the legal concerns raised by government pronouncements, moreover, many authorities opted for indirect rather than direct payments until the legal position was clarified in 1996.

In 1999-2000, the Scottish Executive commissioned Scottish Human Services to investigate the implementation of direct payments in Scotland, with expert input from the Lothian Centre for Independent Living. By combining a telephone survey of 31 Scottish authorities with in-depth interviews with service users, social workers and managers in four case study authorities, the study identified considerable confusion among local authorities about what direct payments are and how they operate (Witcher et al, 2000). Some authorities were unsure about the precise differences between direct and indirect payments, and only 13 (less than half the authorities in Scotland) were making direct payments to disabled people. Altogether, there were 143 people across the

Box 26: 1968 Social Work (Scotland) Act

It shall be the duty of every local authority to promote social welfare ... and ... to provide or secure the provision of such facilities ... as they may consider suitable and adequate, and such assistance may be given to, or in respect of, the persons specified in the next following subsection *in kind or in cash*...

The persons specified for the purposes of the foregoing subsection are:

(a) a person, being a child under the age of eighteen, requiring assistance in kind, or in exceptional circumstances, in cash....

(b) a person in need requiring assistance in kind, or in *exceptional circumstances constituting an emergency*, in cash, where the giving of assistance in either form would *avoid the local authority being caused greater expense* in the giving of assistance in another form, or where probable aggravation of the person's need would cause greater expense to the local authority on a later occasion. (1968 Social Work (Scotland) Act, section 12; emphasis added) whole of Scotland receiving direct payments: 125 (87%) with a physical or sensory impairment, 17 (12%) with a learning difficulty and one person with Asperger's Syndrome. There were no recipients with mental health problems and no users from a minority ethnic group. While some authorities made information about direct payments available, the emphasis was on informing staff rather than informing potential recipients. In some cases, authorities had decided not to publicise direct payments for fear of creating increased demand which the authority might not be able to meet. Five authorities had introduced their own eligibility criteria above and beyond those set out in legislation, targeting people in 'high priority' groups (often defined as being at risk of entering residential care).

Although support schemes were often available, these varied considerably in form and scope and there were concerns about possible gaps in support, particularly for people with learning difficulties. Funding was also very varied and was often hindered by a lack of flexibility between budgets. Payments to individuals ranged from £153 to £4,583 per month, with hourly rates for PAs ranging from £3.60 to £11.64. While some payments included employers' costs and contingency funds, many did not. Recruiting workers was difficult in most authorities, particularly in rural areas. While most authorities were positive about the principles of direct payments, they expressed significant concerns about the practicalities of running direct payment schemes, such as:

- lack of funding to operate schemes;
- a perceived threat to the funding or future of local authority services;
- anxiety about perceived implications for the role of social workers;
- anxiety about some people's ability to manage payments;
- lack of adequate support for recipients.

As a result of this study, further research is planned to investigate the barriers to direct payments for people with mental health problems in Scotland (Scottish Executive Central Research Unit, 2001) and a number of steps are being taken to promote direct payments more widely (see Chapter Four).

Northern Ireland

With no history of third party indirect payments in Northern Ireland (Campbell, nd), progress has been slower than in other parts of the UK. Initially, the implementation of direct payments was delayed for a year due to lack of interest and to enable service providers to prepare for the new system (Valois, 1997). According to one commentator, disability organisations were at least partly to blame since they were largely unaware of direct payments and had not pushed for them (Valois, 1997). Although the Department of Health, Social Services and Public Safety (DHSSPS) has stated that statistics concerning the take-up of direct payments cannot be released for this book (personal communication, DHSSPS), anecdotal evidence suggests that progress has been extremely slow with payments once again confined primarily to people with physical impairments.

Emerging issues in the UK

Despite early enthusiasm and despite the ongoing contribution of a number of key authorities, the implementation of direct payments has been uneven. While some authorities have welcomed the 1996 Act and sought to publicise their direct payments schemes, others have been more reluctant and progress has sometimes been slow. Although direct payments are still a relatively recent phenomenon, both research and anecdotal evidence have revealed a number of barriers to the implementation of direct payments. In Northern Ireland, we have seen how a lack of awareness and a lack of pressure from disability organisations delayed the advent of direct payments (Valois, 1997). Elsewhere, it has been suggested that low take-up in Northern England/Scotland may be because the stronger culture of municipal welfare in traditional Labour areas is less open to empowering service users (McCurry, 1999). For one commentator, such ideological concerns may be creating something of a "north–south divide" (Pearson, 2000, p 463), with Northern English and Scottish authorities perceiving direct payments as a means of eroding public sector service provision, and Conservative-led authorities in Southern England promoting direct payments as a means of encouraging individual choice and cost-efficiency. Other key issues have included a lack of support for the recipients of direct payments as well as a lack of awareness among social workers and a lack of accessible information (see Box 27). In some cases, this is felt to be the result of a lack of pump-priming to establish an appropriate support infrastructure for direct payment schemes (Wellard, 1999).

Even where disabled people have been able to benefit from direct payment schemes, some projects have been introduced on a pilot basis only and leave

Box 27: Barriers to wider implementation of direct payments

- Confusion in some local authorities about what constitutes direct payments
- Perceived need on the part of local authorities to limit demand
- Demands on care managers' time
- Absence of operational infrastructure for direct payments within local authorities
- Lack of information and publicity
- Lack of active recruitment policies, or restrictive recruitment policies
- The national 'ban' on direct payments to older people (now removed)
- The national 'ban' on employing relatives as PAs
- The application of additional and restrictive local criteria
- Funding restraints
- The fact that direct payments are discretionary rather than rights-based and mandatory

(Witcher et al, 2000)

recipients unsure about the future availability of payments. In some cases, there is a suggestion that such 'pilots' are being used as a delaying tactic by local authorities that do not feel that they have the funding or the skills to introduce direct payment schemes. In particular, NCIL identifies four main problems:

- Few 'pilots' have timescales as to when they will end or when they will be reviewed.
- Many disabled people have been refused payments until the 'pilot' is complete, thereby creating waiting lists.
- Many 'pilots' are restricted to people with physical impairments.
- Most 'pilots' have no terms of reference nor any criteria for judging their success/failure (NCIL, ndb, pp 4-5).

European lessons

Outside the UK, many European countries now offer some form of payment scheme whereby disabled people can receive money instead of directly provided services (see Boxes 28 and 29). In Holland, for example, older people are permitted to receive personal budgets with which to purchase care (Pijl, 1997, 2000; Coolen and Weekers, 1998; Weekers and Pijl, 1998). These were piloted on an experimental basis in 1991, evaluated and formally introduced in 1995. Despite pressure from service users, implementation has been slow and personal budgets account for only 3% to 5% of the total care budget. To prevent fraud, recipients control the selection of providers, but money is administered by an intermediary body. In seeking to introduce personal budgets, a number of barriers have been identified (Coolen and Weekers, 1998, pp 54, 58):

- financial barriers (the concern to contain costs);
- social barriers (problems relating to the employment rights of care-givers);
- implementation barriers (difficulty of matching personal budgets to assessments);
- professional opposition (from trades unions and formal service providers).

Box 28: Examples of European direct payments legislation

- 1993 Federal Law on Direct Payments, Austria
- 1998 Social Services Act, Denmark
- 1993 Social Welfare Act and Decree on Support for Informal Care, Finland
- 1997 Special Benefit for Dependent Persons at Home, France
- 1995 Care Insurance Act, Germany
- Provisions Act for Disabled and Elderly People, Netherlands
- 1994 Support and Service Act, Sweden
- 1996 Community Care (Direct Payments) Act, UK
- Personal Assistance Budget (experimental), Belgium
- Law on Social Assistance, Integration and Disabled People, Italy, 1992

(Halloran, 1998)

Box 29: Key features of direct payment schemes: ENIL seminar, 1997

UK: Direct payments were legalised in April 1997 and are discretionary. At the time of the seminar (1997), the scheme excluded people aged 65 and over.

Belgium: A pilot independent living project will begin in July 1997 for 15 people. The scope for employing PAs at antisocial times is limited due to strict legislation and a strong trades union movement.

The Netherlands: Direct payments were introduced in July 1995 for housekeeping, sophisticated housekeeping, personal care and registered nursing services provided in the home, although there was strong opposition from trades unions and government concerns about the potential for abuse.

Austria: Direct payments were available from July 1993, although payments are low and it is expected that people needing more than four hours of care a day will live in an institution.

Germany:The German direct payments system is very medicalised and disabled people receive less money if they choose to receive money directly rather than selecting support from approved providers.

Finland: Personal assistance is available in Finland, although there have been calls to promote this option further as a means of reducing the unemployment level within the disabled community. Payments are made directly to the PA, not through the individual disabled person.

The Czech Republic: Personal assistance was introduced in 1991 and a Centre for Independent Living was established in 1993. In 1997, there were 110 PA users, 60 in Prague and 50 in Allamons. This was possible as there was a disabled civil servant in this municipality.

Norway: Personal assistance can be claimed through the social security system (with payments made via local government, via the user or via cooperatives).

Sweden: Personal assistance has been a right in Sweden since 1994. Users can receive such personal assistance in a range of ways, including as an individual, through a cooperative, with an assistance company and through the municipal services. Due to financial problems, restrictions are being considered.

Bratislava: Direct payments were introduced in January 1997 for an initial group of 21 users.

(ENIL, 1997)

Elsewhere, the form and scope of direct payments vary considerably. In Sweden, disabled people have had a legal right since 1994 to receive personal assistance and to choose their carer or employ them directly. This can include family members and there are around 43,000 participants in the scheme (Wellard, 1999). Under the German social insurance model, eligibility is determined by medical assessment and allowances are calculated on the basis of a pre-set national table of need and cost per hour (Halloran, 1998; Wellard, 1999). Whereas Germany, France and Denmark enable recipients of direct payments to choose services from approved providers, the Scandinavian countries tend to issue vouchers. Although the UK and Denmark provide individual service users with cash payments, disabled people in France, Germany Austria and the Netherlands who opt for such payments receive a smaller sum than the 'in kind' value of services they could receive if they nominated an approved provider (Halloran, 1998).

Overall, research commissioned by the European Association for Care and Help at Home (EACHH) suggests that the shift towards cash payments is the result of a series of parallel developments:

- the growing demand for care and the fact that available care cannot meet new needs;
- pressure, especially from organisations of disabled people;
- new ideology of a care market, which will produce cheaper and better services;
- political wish to let people stay longer in their own homes instead of more expensive institutions;
- a wish to stimulate care provision by informal carers (Pijl, 2000, p 56).

Despite considerable variations between different countries, the EACHH study found that the same key questions were being asked in most countries:

- Will more people apply for cash than for services?
- Should allowances become part of a social insurance system or should it be social assistance?
- What is the best way to assess an applicant and to determine the amount to be paid?
- Will the recipients of cash use it properly?
- Will the quality of services bought with the cash be adequate?
- Will the PAs be treated well by their employees? (Pijl, 2000, pp 56-7)

Ultimately, the EACHH researchers concluded that direct payments were a positive development, but sounded a note of warning:

> Care allowances, a new device, are practical and useful for certain categories of people. Those who can handle the responsibilities are, as a rule, positive about this innovation. For those who receive a care allowance it is important to have recourse, either to an informal network or a formal agency to help when there are problems. I think care allowances are not a good way of

> helping very frail or confused and isolated people who live by themselves. Care allowances may serve to reduce the visibility of the needs of these people who are no longer able to speak up for themselves. Who is responsible in our individualised and marketised societies for these people who have lost both their autonomy and their social network? (Pijl, 2000, p 64)

SUMMARY

Introduced on a discretionary rather than a mandatory basis, the progress of direct payments has often been extremely slow, with different local authorities adopting different approaches. In general, implementation has been much more rapid in the south of England than in the north, Wales, Northern Ireland and many parts of Scotland. Key barriers to the spread of direct payments appear to include fears about the erosion of public services, a lack of awareness among social workers, financial concerns, a lack of accessible information and the absence of pump-priming to establish appropriate support mechanisms. Despite these barriers, direct payments have also been introduced in a number of European countries (with the UK implementing payments much later than some of its neighbours). While a variety of approaches have been adopted and while many countries are struggling with obstacles to further progress, the fact that payments are available in so many different countries suggests that the concept of direct payments may well be an idea whose time has come.

SIX

The experiences of different user groups

The strongest calls for direct payments to be introduced came from organisations of disabled people, many of whom had previously benefited from the choice and control offered by indirect payments and the ILF (Kestenbaum, 1993a, 1993b, 1999; Morris, 1993a). As a result, direct payments have tended to be associated primarily with people with physical impairments, and many of the advantages cited in Chapter Seven of this book are often advantages described from the perspective of people with physical impairments or their representatives. In contrast, research to date suggests that relatively few people with learning difficulties have been offered the opportunity to receive direct payments, with even fewer recipients among people with mental health problems, older people and people with HIV/AIDS. Direct payments have also been shown to raise particular issues for people from minority ethnic groups and for gay men/ lesbians. Against this background, this chapter explores the different experiences of various user groups, considering issues such as access to direct payments, the attitudes of practitioners and possible ways forward.

People with physical impairments

Throughout the UK, the vast majority of people receiving direct payments have been those classed as having physical impairments. In 1998, Department of Health research suggested that 1,329 of 1,404 direct payment recipients in England (95%) were people with physical or sensory impairments (Auld, 1999). By 2000, the ADSS found that 110 out of 136 English and Welsh authorities had direct payment schemes available to service users with all types of impairment, but noted that a significant minority excluded particular groups of people (Jones, 2000). In Scotland, 87% of recipients of direct payments have physical or sensory impairments (Witcher et al, 2000).

In many ways, this should not be surprising, since people with physical impairments have traditionally formed user groups that have been more powerful and politically active than those of other service users (M. Barnes, 1997). At the same time, the imperative to ensure that recipients of direct payments are willing and able to manage them (alone or with assistance) is likely to have been interpreted by some local authorities as ruling out most user groups other than people with physical impairments. In some locations, staff specialising in work with people with physical impairments may also be much more familiar with the concepts of independent living and direct payments than their colleagues in mental health, learning difficulty or other teams. Certainly this seems to have been the case in one evaluation of a direct payments scheme, which found that take-up was higher among people with physical impairments than for other user groups (Dawson, 2000). This was the result of a number of factors:

- The local direct payments scheme prevented payments for services such as day care, while government regulations prevented the use of direct payments for residential care. This excluded many people with mental health problems or learning difficulties, since day and residential care were especially common for these user groups.
- Staff involved in the direct payments project came from physical impairment teams.
- Documentation concerning direct payments was ambiguously worded and was not sent to the managers of mental health or learning difficulty teams.
- Staff working with people with physical impairments were more likely to be aware of a previous indirect payment project and to be familiar with the concept of users employing their own PAs.
- There was a widespread assumption that people with learning difficulties and mental health problems would not be able to manage direct payments.
- A local coalition of disabled people represented a range of user groups, but was dominated by people with physical impairments.
- The direct payments coordinator employed by the coalition moved from working at home to an office in a day centre which traditionally served people with physical impairments.

In recognition of the need to make direct payments available for people other than those with physical impairments, the government has acted to ensure that people from different user groups are not excluded from existing schemes. In 2000, revised guidance emphasised that suitability for direct payments must be assessed on a case-by-case basis, with no blanket exclusions of any user groups

Box 30: Including all user groups

Local authorities need to satisfy themselves that the scheme they develop serves all adult client groups equitably... When deciding upon whether to offer Direct Payments to a person authorities should take care not to fetter their discretion. An authority cannot make a decision covering all cases: it must consider each individual case.

Local authorities have the discretion to refuse direct payments to anyone who they judge would not (with appropriate support) be able to manage them, but should avoid making blanket assumptions that whole groups of people will necessarily be unable to do so. The judgement as to whether someone is able to manage will need to be made on an individual basis, taking into account the views of the individual himself or herself. (DoH, 2000a, pp 4, 15) (see Box 30). This was underlined by Health Minister, John Hutton, who stated that "more needs to be done to ensure the benefits of independent living are available to people with learning disabilities, mental illness and HIV/AIDS. Every local authority in the country needs to be aware that they must not fetter their discretion in deciding who should get direct payments" (quoted in Hasler, 1999, p 7). Of course the larger numbers of people with physical impairments who receive direct payments should not be seen as problematic in itself and can clearly be viewed as evidence of significant progress. As a result, the aim should not be to reduce the number of people with physical impairments who receive direct payments, but to increase the number of people from other user groups who may face particular barriers to existing payment schemes.

Despite the orientation of direct payments towards people with physical impairments, there are particular groups of people whose experiences of direct payments are less well documented. Thus, there seems too little emphasis in the literature on people with specific impairments (such as acquired brain injuries or cerebral palsy), who may face barriers similar to those described below for people with learning difficulties or mental health problems. Another key group whose needs are often overlooked is disabled parents, who may require additional hours as part of a direct payments care package for the physical aspects of parenting (see Box 31). Such people clearly face additional demands and pressures as direct payment recipients, since they are responsible not only for their own care, but also for the welfare of dependent children (Dawson, 2000). In one study, disabled parents were acutely aware of these responsibilities, and felt that direct payments could offer them the control and flexibility they needed to raise their family as they saw fit (Dawson, 2000). Elsewhere, some social services departments may not be so responsive to the needs of disabled parents. A Department of Health (1998c) promotional video shows a woman with a visual impairment who receives a direct payment to assist her with looking after a child, but there have also been cases where an authority has suggested that it would be more cost-effective to foster a new baby than enable the disabled parent to care for their own child through direct payments (Hasler et al, 1999, p 33). Funding can also be difficult, since it can fall between the remit of children's teams and adult services. Although concerns have been raised about the safety of children in households that employ a PA, some commentators emphasise that the solution is simply for the parent to

Box 31: Disabled parents

"It's been really good for us as a family. My husband has been able to go back to work since I started getting direct payments, because he wasn't having to do all the housework and looking after the children. Also, my own health has improved because I am less tired all the time struggling to do things I really wasn't capable of. I have good days and bad days and services did not offer what I needed, you either have them or you don't, they come at set times. With this, I use it as and when I need it. This scheme has transformed the quality of life for us as a family." (quoted in Hasler et al, 1999, p 34) employ a trustworthy person (Hasler et al, 1999). More recently, safety issues have been addressed in more detail following the 2000 Carers and Disabled Children Act (see Chapter Four).

In 1998-99, a Social Services Inspectorate report into services to support disabled parents found that this user group was sometimes excluded from direct payment schemes (Goodinge, 2000). Although many disabled parents were positive about direct payments and felt that this may help to meet their parenting needs, few parents were receiving payments. This was the result of four main factors:

- numbers of direct payment recipients were low overall;
- schemes were not well publicised;
- parenting needs were rarely assessed and could not therefore be part of a direct payments package;
- many staff were unclear about the usefulness of direct payments and whether parenting needs should be part of community care (Goodinge, 2000, p 22).

People with learning difficulties

When the Community Care (Direct Payments) Bill was being debated, the government's initial intention was to restrict direct payments to people with physical impairments until the new scheme could be tested in practice (see Chapter Three and DoH/Scottish Office/Welsh Office/Northern Ireland Office, 1996). While people with both a physical impairment and learning difficulties might have been eligible for direct payments, people with learning difficulties alone would have been excluded, at least in the early years of the new scheme. This restriction was eventually overturned following concerted lobbying by organisations such as People First, and subsequent policy and practice guidance has emphasised that local authorities should avoid blanket assumptions that whole groups of people are unable manage payments (DoH, 1997a, 2000a). Despite this, people with learning difficulties continue to experience a number of barriers to receiving direct payments, both in terms of practical issues raised by the way in which direct payments have been implemented, and in terms of prejudicial attitudes within local authorities and central government.

In 1997, a Social Services Inspectorate report into services for adults with learning difficulties found that only one of the eight authorities inspected was actively considering a direct payments scheme for this user group (Fruin, 1998). By 1999, an inspection into independent living arrangements for younger disabled people found that some authorities were inappropriately excluding entire user groups from direct payment schemes (Fruin, 2000). In some areas, this included people with learning difficulties, who were sometimes felt to require additional, and potentially costly, support arrangements. In Scotland, research suggests that there are only 17 people with a learning difficulty receiving direct payments (12% of all recipients) (Witcher et al, 2000). In north-west England, research carried out by the North West Training and Development

Team (NWTDT) in 1998 suggested that the vast majority of social services departments were moving only tentatively towards direct payments and that many had no plans to extend direct payments to people with learning difficulties (Gardner, 1999).

Throughout England as a whole, Department of Health statistics reveal that on 30 September 1998 there were 39 people with learning difficulties (under 3% of all recipients) receiving direct payments and that these people were spread across a mere eight local authorities (Auld, 1999). Of these, three people were from the central region, four were from London, 19 were from the northern region and 11 were from the southern region. Crucially, these numbers had begun to increase from previous monitoring and, rather than comment on the low numbers of people with learning difficulties receiving direct payments, the Department of Health chose to portray this increase as evidence of progress. In autumn 2000, the number of people with learning difficulties receiving direct payments had risen to 216 out of a total of over 3,700 (less than 6%) (DoH, 2001f, p 48). By 2001, government rhetoric had begun to change, with a new White Paper on services for people with learning difficulties acknowledging that this user group had all too often been excluded from direct payment schemes (DoH, 2001f, p 48). In a one-page section on direct payments, the government states:

- People with learning difficulties can benefit from the increased choice and control which direct payments bring.
- The small number of people with learning difficulties receiving direct payments is unacceptable.
- The provisions of the Health and Social Care Act are intended to result in more people with learning difficulties receiving direct payments.
- The success of direct payments for people with learning difficulties depends on good support services. Since many local authority support schemes focus on people with physical impairments, the government will issue guidance under the Health and Social Care Act so that people with learning difficulties can be assisted to use direct payments.
- The Implementation Support Team (a national team promoting good practice in services for people with learning difficulties) will work with local councils to ensure a higher take-up of direct payments.
- The Department of Health will consult on a performance indicator in the Personal Social Services Performance Assessment Framework.

Despite government pressure to increase access to direct payments for people with learning difficulties, however, a number of barriers to participation remain. Throughout the literature, a recurring theme is the insistence of Department of Health guidance (1997a) that direct payment recipients are *willing and able* to manage the money they receive, either alone or with assistance. This has caused significant confusion for many local authorities, raising complex legal issues and challenging professional dilemmas about capacity and how best to assess people's ability to make decisions for themselves (see Bewley, 1998; Holman and Bewley, 1999; Ryan and Holman, 1999a for a more detailed discussion). While some authorities have responded by excluding people with learning difficulties from their direct payment schemes, others are less concerned about people's ability to consent as long as direct payments are working successfully for individual recipients (Ryan and Holman, 1999a). Although few local authorities may admit to this in public, practitioners and policy makers at both a local and central level have privately suggested that they overlook the technicalities of ability and consent in situations where they feel that direct payments are the best option for service users (personal communications). Change may also be underway in Scotland where there are proposals to extend direct payments to guardians/attorneys on behalf of people unable to manage their own payments (see Chapter Four and Scottish Executive, 2001).

In addressing issues of consent and capacity, several commentators have suggested ways forward for service users and practitioners alike. One solution is for money to be paid to people with learning difficulties via a trust fund (see Holman, 1995 for a sample trust deed) or for service users to receive support from an independent advocate or from a microboard (see Box 32).

Box 32: Microboards

Developed initially in Canada, Microboards are to be piloted in Northern Ireland for a family who had previously moved to the province from Canada:

> A Microboard is a small, closely connected group of family and friends that form a friendship circle with a person who has a learning difficulty. Microboards also operate as not-for-profit groups. Each Microboard is created to support one person. They plan with the person to create a unique and intimate support service. The person for whom the Microboard is created drives the direction their board will take. Each Microboard is different, reflecting the person's own interests, beliefs, and individualised support needs. The Microboard members make a commitment to be part of the individual's personal network, introducing them to and ensuring they are included in their community. Microboards also contract with appropriate funding agencies to provide individualised funding and service supports for the person for whom the board has been created.... For those people with learning difficulties, who may not be able to manage the day-to-day supervision of their services, Microboards are a way of remaining at the centre of their support, and in control, but with the additional help they need. (Holman and Bewley, 1999, pp 66-7)

To clarify the complex professional judgements which the *willing and able* guidance necessitates, researchers evaluating the implementation of a direct payments scheme in Norfolk have also developed a checklist for social workers seeking to assess an individual's capacity to make decisions (Dawson, 2000, Appendix 2; Dawson and McDonald, 2000). Although the checklist includes a range of issues to consider, these are grouped under eight key headings:

- What is the significance of the life history of the person on this decision?
- Is the person able to make a decision?
- What is the significance of a particular decision?
- What is known about the person's ability to communicate?
- Has information been presented in different formats?
- What were the circumstances of the decision making?
- Who was involved in the decision making process?
- How quickly was the decision required?

For Ryan and Holman (1999a, pp 15-20), there are a number of key issues if direct payments are to be accessible to people with learning difficulties:

- Informed consent can only occur when people with learning difficulties are given accessible information.
- Pressure should be minimised by giving people plenty of time to express their preferences and choosing an appropriate environment for any assessment of consent.
- Formal procedures for receiving direct payments should be simplified as much as possible.
- People's preferred method of communication should be respected.
- Significant others should be involved in assessing capacity.
- Person Centred Planning is crucial to the success of direct payments for people with learning difficulties (see also Sanderson and Kilbane, 1999; Routledge and Sanderson, 2000).
- People with learning difficulties should be permitted to take more control over their lives (and therefore take more risks).
- Safeguards should be developed to prevent abuse and monitor risks.
- Direct payments should work in a spirit of partnership between the service user, their family and the local authority.
- Local authorities should not set too many prerequisites for people with learning difficulties before they can access direct payments.
- Local authorities must learn through practice and adopt a problem solving approach.
- Direct payments have been most successful where someone with sufficient power and vision takes a lead role within the local authority.

In addition to the *willing and able* debate, people with learning difficulties have also been excluded from direct payments through a range of other barriers. In many areas of the country, information about direct payments may not be available in accessible formats and members of staff working with people with learning difficulties may not be aware of direct payments themselves (Holman and Bewley, 1999). Certainly, this was the case in a study in Tower Hamlets, where, out of a group of 10 people with learning difficulties, 10 members of staff and 10 carers, only two members of staff had heard of direct payments (Maglajlic et al, 2000, pp 100-1; see also Chapter Eight). At the same time, some social workers may be withholding information about direct payments from people with learning difficulties in situations where the worker feels that the user will be unable to manage (Dawson, 2000). While staff believed that it was unreasonable to raise a service user's hopes unnecessarily, the researcher in this particular study felt that practitioners may be working on the basis of discriminatory assumptions about people with learning difficulties, not on the results of an individual and objective assessment (Dawson, 2000).

To overcome the barriers to direct payments which people with learning difficulties have faced, the Department of Health (2000b) has developed *An easy guide to direct payments* in conjunction with Values Into Action (VIA) (see page 71) and the Informability Unit at the Central Office of Information. To make direct payments as accessible to as many people as possible, the guide is available free of charge, is written in large print, contains a large range of colour photographs and pictures to support the text and is accompanied by an audio tape and CD. The guide explains the nature of direct payments, how to access this option, how the money can be spent, how to set up and manage a payment scheme and how to get further information. Crucially, the guide emphasises two key features about direct payments: "you are in control; they [social services departments] are not in control" (DoH, 2000b, pp 7-9). Building on previous policy and practice guidance (DoH, 1997a), the guide is also very explicit that social services departments cannot exclude whole groups of people from direct payments on the basis of assumptions about their ability to manage payments: "Social Services ... cannot say that they do not give Direct Payments to people with learning disabilities" (DoH, 2000b, p 10).

In addition to this official guidance, a number of organisations have been involved in developing materials for people with learning difficulties and exploring the issues which direct payments raise for this user group. In 1998, Changing Perspectives and NCIL developed a training pack "to help people think about the issues involved in assessing a user's ability to manage direct payments" (Aspis, 1998, p 1). The pack is designed to be photocopied onto overhead projector slides and handouts, using a series of illustrations and images to cover topics such as:

- what life is like for many disabled people;
- a day in the life of a disabled person using social services;
- what life could be like for a disabled person able to buy their own support;
- a day in the life of a disabled person using direct payments;
- the things that disable disabled people;
- barriers to being assessed for ability to manage direct payments;
- suggested questions for assessments.

In addition to the work of Changing Perspectives/NCIL, the Royal College of Nursing's Learning Disability Nursing Forum held a facilitated discussion among delegates at one of its conferences (Francis, 2001). During the discussion, many participants expressed their concern about the low take-up of direct payments among people with learning difficulties, the limited nature of available information, the tightening of local authority eligibility criteria due to financial restrictions and the lack of clarity within local authorities about direct payments and the interface with ILF payments. While the results of this conference have only been written up as a short introductory article (Francis, 2001), the involvement of learning disability nurses in debates about direct payments is an important step forward, particularly in light of the issues which direct payments raise for the health and social care divide (see Chapters Seven and Eight).

Probably the largest body of literature on direct payments and people with learning difficulties has been produced by VIA, a campaigning organisation committed to changing laws, services and attitudes so that people with learning difficulties can become valued citizens. Under the overall heading *Funding freedom*, VIA has undertaken a series of projects on the use of direct payments by people with learning difficulties. This includes national conferences, research and guidance on the implementation and development of the Direct Payments Act (Holman and Collins, 1997), a briefing paper on supported decision making (Bewley, 1998) and video and audio cassettes (Holman, 1998a, 1998b). More

Box 33: Making direct payments happen for people with learning disabilities

A joint programme by the North West Training and Development Team (NWTDT) and Values Into Action, September 2000–April 2001

Take-up of direct payments by people with learning disabilities has been disappointingly slow... This programme aims to provide information and practical support to departments serious about making direct payments happen for people with learning disabilities. It is clear to us that introducing direct payments requires both technical knowledge and skills and planning around introducing innovation....

There are two options:

Option 1 will offer:

- Access to the latest information from around the country/networking about effective approaches to introducing direct payments for people with learning disabilities.
- Facilitated action planning for district teams working to introduce or develop direct payments.
- Access to expert information and advice between formal sessions.
- The opportunity to network with other people serious about implementing direct payments.
- Preferential and substantially reduced price access to NWTDT Managing Change programme ... to support change activity around direct payments...
- Each team will receive 11 days of input over 7 months, plus telephone/email advice as needed.

Option 2 offers the above input minus team participation on the Managing Change course. (NWTDT, 2000a) recently, VIA has employed a presenter to explain direct payments to self-advocacy groups around the country, supported the development of direct payments in Scotland (Henderson and Bewley, 2000) and worked with local authorities to guide the implementation of direct payments for people with learning difficulties (see Box 33). Drawing on this experience, VIA has launched its *Funding freedom 2000* report (Holman and Bewley, 1999), summarising the findings of its various projects.

Also significant in the campaign to improve access to direct payments for people with learning difficulties has been *Community Living*, an independent journal devoted to working for a fully inclusive society for people with learning difficulties. Both during, and after, the campaign for direct payments, *Community*

Box 34: An ode to direct payments

A carer who's a stranger, comes knocking at my door
Having to explain my needs, I've done this all before
The plates are in that cupboard, and the spoons are over here
The Hoover's in the other room; and here's the cleaning gear.

You get to know your carer and they get to know you,
And then you have to start again, because it's someone new.
Embarrassing for all of us, as personal needs described
My privacy and dignity to some degree denied!

But now there's an alternative for the provision of my care
I can become an employer and choose who I want there.
They call it 'Direct payments' it offers more control
Disenchanted individuals, this scheme may well console.

At first it seems quite daunting, as with most things that are new.
Can the 'Darlington Direct Payment Scheme' really work for you?
Peer support is offered by some who use this scheme
Developing my confidence and heightening self-esteem.

My Personal Assistants are people of my choosing
At first I found the paperwork a little bit confusing!
The Direct Payment Support Service assisting whilst it's needed
Another Direct Payment user, who can say they have succeeded.

Of course it won't suit everyone, but now we have a choice
There really is no pressure, your preference given voice
And should you wish to try the scheme, then find it's not for you
Your previous care arrangements, resumed without ado.

(Taylor, 2000, p 7)

Living has published a constant stream of articles, commentaries and information sheets, and hardly an edition goes by without at least some mention of direct payments and independent living issues (see, for example, Box 34).

Despite growing awareness of the potential which direct payments may have for people with learning difficulties, however, the fact remains that current government guidance and its explicit emphasis on being *willing and able* to manage payments is likely to continue to act as a barrier for people with learning difficulties. This is a clear example of the way in which direct payments (in their current form) have been conceptualised and implemented from a physical impairment perspective without taking adequate account of the needs of people with learning difficulties. Until government guidance changes, it is unlikely that the low take-up by people with learning difficulties will change much either.

People with mental health problems

In contrast to the experience of people with physical impairments and with learning difficulties, the experience of people with mental health problems has often been overlooked and, with some notable exceptions, the accessibility of direct payments has rarely been discussed. This neglect of mental health issues was immediately apparent during the initial implementation of direct payments, when the 1996 consultation paper on the Direct Payments Bill made no reference to the needs of people with mental health problems at all (except for excluding certain groups of people detained under mental health legislation). Although the government suggested that direct payments might be made available to people with a physical impairments and another condition (such as a learning disability), there seemed to be no recognition that "another condition" could include mental health problems, or that people with mental health problems without a physical impairment might benefit from direct payments (DoH/ Scottish Office/Welsh Office/Northern Ireland Office, 1996, p 4). As the Direct Payments Bill was being debated in Parliament, moreover, there were specific attempts to exclude all service users with mental health problems (Beresford, 1996). Even after the 1997 policy and practice guidance was issued (DoH, 1997a), there were very few references to people with mental health problems in the documentation and no recognition at all that they might face additional barriers to direct payments. Nor has this been rectified in the revised 2000 policy and practice guidance (DoH, 2000a), which is no more sensitive to the needs of people with mental health problems than the document it replaced.

In light of this neglect in the official literature, it is hardly surprising that people with mental health problems have often found it difficult to access direct payments. Although it is difficult to be specific, it has been estimated that at one stage only 10 people with mental problems were receiving direct payments throughout the UK (Maglajlic, 1999; Revans, 2000), with no direct payment recipients with mental health problems in Scotland at all (Witcher et al, 2000). As a result, the Scottish Executive has sought to commission new research to investigate the barriers to direct payments for people with mental health problems (Scottish Executive Central Research Unit, 2001). By 30 September 1998, the number of mental health service users receiving direct payment in England had risen to 13, spread over seven social services departments (Auld, 1999). With four such direct payment recipients, Essex was identified as one of the leading authorities (Brandon, 1998; Revans, 2000). Outside the UK, very few countries have developed widespread direct payment schemes for people with mental health problems; with one commentator suggesting that Alberta in Canada is one of the only places in the world to use direct payments in a significant fashion for people coming out of 'mental hospitals' (Brandon, 1998). Ironically, it appears as though the small number of British direct payment recipients with mental health problems (most of them concentrated in Essex) places Britain ahead of many of its European neighbours:

> In one small area of one small county – Essex – seem to live most of the people in Europe who are mental health users accessing direct payments. Our heartfelt congratulations to them. (Brandon, 1998, p 26)

Although there is very little literature on direct payments and mental health, research undertaken by Anglia Polytechnic University (Brandon, 1998; Maglajlic, 1999; Maglajlic et al, 1998, 2000) and a number of important commentaries/testimonies (Irish, 1998; Luckhurst, 2000; NCIL, ndc; Revans, 2000) have begun to identify some key issues. In May 1997, a study began in Tower Hamlets, London involving three user groups – people with learning difficulties, people with physical impairments and people with mental health problems (Maglajlic, 1999; Maglajlic et al, 1998, 2000). With each user group, semi-structured interviews were conducted with 10 service users, 10 staff and 10 carers. For people with mental health problems, the main barriers to receiving direct payments included (Maglajlic, 1999; Maglajlic et al, 1998):

- A lack of knowledge about direct payments among service users, staff and carers.
- Low expectations of social services due to previous poor experiences.
- High eligibility criteria for access to social services, with some service users feeling that they had to be almost 'sectionable' before they received any support.
- Difficulties managing money when ill and an awareness of being perceived as people not trusted to take care of themselves. For direct payments to be successful, all users and carers felt that they would need support, particularly when handling money and recruiting staff.
- The lack of other mental health service users using direct payments elsewhere.

In 2000, many of these issues were re-emphasised by a commentary in *Community Care* (Revans, 2000). Drawing on interviews with representatives from a number of independent living projects, key issues for people with mental health problems were felt to include the emphasis of the 1996 Act on the needs of people with physical impairments coupled with "the varying degrees of ignorance, anxiety and reluctance displayed by local authorities" (Revans, 2000, p 12). Also significant was the tendency for people with mental health problems to have much more contact with health professionals such as community psychiatric nurses than with social services departments.

Despite all these barriers, participating service users in the Tower Hamlets study felt that direct payments might enable them to obtain flexible support at home/in the evenings/at weekends, to access community activities and to maintain employment/return to work. A particularly striking example of the benefits of direct payments for people with mental health problems comes from the testimony of a direct payment recipient living in a small village in Essex (Irish, 1998). After negative experiences with health and social care workers and adverse drug reactions, Hazel Irish (not her real name) describes how she was "virtually a zombie", unable to get out of bed, wash or dress by herself (Irish, 1998, p 28). After beginning to receive direct payments, she began to get help with cleaning her home and getting out of the house. Despite excessive interference from her social worker and difficulties persuading agency workers to visit such a remote area, Hazel feels that direct payments are a major step forward (see Box 35).

Accounts such as that of Hazel are a major testimony to the ability of direct payments to transform the lives of people who have been previously disempowered and who have not been able to obtain a satisfactory response to their needs from directly provided statutory services. Against this background, it is to be deeply regretted that so few people with mental health problems have been enabled to access direct payments. At the time of the Tower Hamlets study, the researchers were only aware of four people with mental health problems receiving direct payments in the whole of the country and concluded their work with an urgent plea for an extension of payments to a larger number of people:

> There will not be an un-manageable demand for direct payments. The majority still doesn't know they exist. Their expectations of services in general are too low. Even with necessary, flexible support organised according to levels identified by users as needed, this will be a gradual process. But it is one that more than four people have a right to. (Maglajlic et al, 1998, pp 42-3)

Box 35: Direct payments and mental health

"I benefit a lot from Direct Payments. The idea of getting cash you can control is brilliant.... Instead of a social worker or nurse dictating what I can and cannot do, it gives me real control. If I'm going to get back to being me again, I can't achieve that with someone bossing me about.... I'll fight to get more control over my life. Now that I have more energy and can think more clearly I want to direct what happens to me more and more." (Irish, 1998, p 32)

More recently, NCIL has published a guide to direct payments for people with mental health problems (NCIL, ndc). Available via the NCIL website (see the Appendix), the guide begins with introductory information about the nature and practicalities of direct payments before moving on to address issues specific to users of mental health services. This includes ways in which service users can continue to manage their payments if they become unwell, such as advance directives (for example, what a support worker should do in particular circumstances, such as a crisis) or user-controlled trusts. Other key issues include safety and risk, insurance, training, obtaining flexible support as needs change and confidentiality. Finally, the guide concludes with details of useful organisations, websites and publications.

In addition to the NCIL guidance, the Institute for Applied Health and Social Policy at King's College London is in the process of developing a three-year pilot scheme to promote direct payments for people with mental health problems in five sites in England (Hampshire, Surrey, Barnet, Leicester and Greater Manchester). At the time of writing, the Institute is preparing a website with contact details for the various pilots and will publish a twice-yearly newsletter (see NCIL, ndc, for further details). Further information on direct payments and mental health is also available from the UK Advocacy Network, which has published two articles on this topic in the May 2001 edition of *The Advocate* newsletter. In the first article, NCIL's Linda Luckhurst (2001) provides introductory information on direct payments and where to go for further information. In the second article, a mental health service user receiving direct payments highlights the strengths and limitations of her payments package (Heslop, 2001). While key advantages include a sense of control, greater confidence/independence and mental health promotion, limitations include the sometimes overwhelming tasks of recruiting, selecting and managing personal assistants, particularly when unwell. Overall, however, the author concludes with an upbeat message about the capacity of direct payments to transform lives and promote independence:

> For all the pitfalls and potential difficulties, the Direct Payments Scheme has given me a life that I could not have envisaged five years ago. It CAN work very effectively with mental health service users, and the assumption that people could not cope because of their diagnostic label needs challenging. I hope that other mental health service users will have the same opportunities as me to use a truly user-centred and user-led option. It is high time that we demanded it as one of a range of all too limited or non-existent choices that are currently available. (Heslop, 2001, p 9)

Older people

When direct payments were first implemented under the 1996 Community Care (Direct Payments) Act, the legislation prohibited payments to people aged 65 or over (unless the person concerned had been receiving such payments

Table 9: Social services expenditure in England (1997-98)

	Older people	Children	Learning difficulties	Physical impairment	Mental health	Other
£ million	4,910	2,260	1,320	700	510	270

Source: Adapted from Hill (2000, p 11)

before the age of 65). This was in keeping with a similar restriction which had previously been placed on the ILF (see Chapter Two) and was widely interpreted as an attempt to prevent the 'floodgates' from opening in terms of public expenditure (Means and Smith, 1998a, p 60). Certainly, older people in the UK are major users of social services. Although estimates vary, it has been suggested that people aged 65 and over may account for some 47% of total public expenditure on health and social care in England (Victor, 1997, p 91), and they are by far and away the biggest single user group (see Table 9). Should direct payments prove a costly experiment, any attempt to extend the scheme to older people would have major implications for public spending.

Despite this, there was widespread concern about the discriminatory nature of the initial direct payments legislation and sustained pressure from organisations such as NCIL and Age Concern to remove the 65 age limit (Age Concern, 1998; NCIL, ndb, 1999; see also Box 36). As a result, the New Labour government announced its intention to extend direct payments to people aged 65 and over (DoH, 1998a), a decision also welcomed by the Royal Commission on Long-

Box 36: Disabled people over 65

NCIL has received a steady stream of requests over the past six months from people over 65 who want to know what can be done to change the Act's age exclusion. This minority felt the existing age limit of 65 to be purely 'age discrimination'. They felt the decision to restrict on the grounds of age was based on an unfounded assumption that the flood gates would open and demand could not be met. In addition they felt that there was also a strong feeling from Social Services Departments and politicians that older people could 'not cope with the responsibilities of managing a Direct Payment'.

Similar arguments to this were put forward to people with various mental or illness related impairments, as an argument for confining the Act to people with physical impairments. These objections were demolished by reasoned debate throughout the passage of the Bill. Experience has shown that the arguments for restriction on the grounds of impairment were nonsensical and that the SSD [social services department] assessment process should be the instrument that gauges whether an individual has the necessary ability to manage a Direct Payment, not a stated list of impairments or age. *In light of this evidence NCIL urges the Government to repeal the age limit (currently below 65) and simply restrict the option to those who are 'able and willing'. Age alone cannot be considered a reasonable measure of one's competency to manage a Direct Payment.* (NCIL, ndb, pp 2-3; emphasis in the original)

Term Care (1999). Following the extension of direct payments to people over 65 in 2000, there is growing speculation as to how older people will experience direct payments. In early 2001, NCIL was aware of some 23 authorities attempting to offer direct payments to older people (personal communication). Once again, one of the leading authorities was Hampshire, which had 40 older people receiving payments – about 10 of whom were already on direct payments and turned 65, 13 of whom transferred from an indirect payment scheme and about 20 of whom were new to the scheme (Valois, 2000a).

To date, the limited research available suggests that older people may face specific barriers to direct payments, but that these can be overcome with the right support (Zarb and Oliver, 1993; C. Barnes, 1997; Hasler et al, 1999). In 1993, the University of Greenwich published research funded by the Joseph Rowntree Foundation, into the experience of ageing with a disability (Zarb and Oliver, 1993). Drawing on interviews and oral/written accounts from around 300 disabled people, the research suggested that independence was a central concern for many older people who felt that this was being threatened by physical decline or by the lack of appropriate support. Many respondents felt that their needs were being overlooked and that the services available served to reinforce rather than combat dependency. In particular, key issues included a lack of information, restricted living options, unmet needs and unresponsive, inflexible services. Despite their frustration with existing social services provision, few respondents were aware that other disabled people recruited and employed their own PAs or that support was available from Centres for Independent Living. Overall, attitudes to PA schemes were mixed. Although very few people were using PAs during the research, one in five suggested that they would do so in the near future and a similar number said that they might consider it if their circumstances changed. Although some participants valued the independence that employing a PA could bring, others were concerned about taking on additional responsibilities (for example, as an employer) or about making significant changes in their lifestyle. Overall, the researchers felt that the "hiring and firing" model of previous indirect payment schemes might not be the best option for older people, but that there was a significant demand for policy measures to enable older people to maintain their independence (Zarb and Oliver, 1993, pp 121-2).

In 1996, Help the Aged commissioned the BCODP Research Unit at Leeds University to carry out research into older people's views on direct payments. Based on focus groups with 60 older people across three case study sites, the research found that most older people knew very little about direct payments and initially found the concept confusing and alarming (C. Barnes, 1997). Particular issues included the fear that receiving direct payments might lead to a reduction in other benefits or services and a widespread sense that direct payments might be just another cost cutting exercise by the government. Participants were also concerned about personal security, the complexity of managing a direct payment and possible liabilities as an employer. Despite this, many people felt that direct payments might be a useful option for younger disabled people and were angry that this option was restricted to people under

65. Possible benefits of direct payments for older people were thought to include maintaining a sense of independence, enhancing choice, achieving better value for money, improving relationships between users and helpers and providing a greater sense of control. Possible limitations to the scheme included regulations preventing the employment of relatives, restrictions on employing friends and neighbours on a casual basis and the danger of exploitation by care agencies seeking to make money out of older people. For direct payments to be appropriate for older people, it was thought that there needed to be appropriate and accessible information and training, the option to employ relatives and friends, national and local registers of paid helpers and help with administration and self-operated support schemes. There was also a strong sense that direct payments should be one of a range of options, with well-resourced services available as a back up.

In 1999, Portsmouth social services department piloted a new scheme for older people which sought to build on the key features of direct payments (Clark and Spafford, 2001a, 2001b). Although payments had not then been extended to older people, Portsmouth offered a range of options for those deemed 'willing and able' to have their care needs met through a PA, an independent sector agency or the local authority. While the department did not make cash available directly to individual service users, participants were able to negotiate when services were to be provided and 'bank' unused hours for future use. After a nine-month pilot, there were 31 older people using the scheme, with 13 managing their own scheme and 18 using carers to manage the care package on their behalf. Of the 31 older people, 20 chose an independent sector provider, four chose local authority home care services and seven chose packages provided by a PA. A subsequent evaluation (Clark and Spafford, 2001a) revealed a number of key themes and tensions:

- Although a small number of older people chose the PA option, these individuals reported receiving high quality services. Barriers to more people taking up this option included concerns about the safety of advertising and a lack of personal contacts to find a suitable worker.
- While some care managers were enthusiastic about the scheme, others felt constrained by workloads and were concerned about how best to convey the scheme to service users.
- The lack of a designated support worker meant that this task often fell to care managers or to carers.
- Only two participants were from a minority ethnic group, and language was a major barrier.
- Some carers saw the scheme as a means to enhance their own choice and control, raising questions as to who was benefiting most from the scheme: service users or their carers.
- Some care managers were unsure about their role in assessing whether someone was 'willing and able' to take part in the scheme.
- The study identified tensions between promoting empowerment versus protecting users against abuse.

Elsewhere, experience suggests that many older people may be unsure about direct payments and may be less inclined to take on the administrative duties of being an employer (Hasler et al, 1999; Hasler and Zarb, 2000). However, there is no reason why these responsibilities could not be dealt with through more structured support options such as block insurance policies, the use of a payroll bureau, advocacy services or care from an independent agency. For direct payments to be successfully extended to older people, a greater proportion of time may also need to be spent as part of the assessment process explaining direct payments, discussing concerns and exploring possible solutions. Above all, NCIL has identified four key factors affecting the successful implementation of direct payments more generally, and believes that these apply equally to older people:

- *outreach:* so people get to know about direct payments
- *local support*
- *enthused and informed care managers:* so that referrals are made for direct payments
- *holistic and realistic community care assessments:* so that care packages are workable (Hasler and Zarb, 2000).

HIV/AIDS

In England in 1998, 13 service users with HIV/AIDS were receiving direct payments spread over seven authorities (four users in London, eight in the north and one in the south) (Auld, 1999). These numbers are too small to comment on with any accuracy, but preliminary work undertaken by NCIL and the National AIDS Trust suggests that direct payments may be a particularly useful option for people with HIV/AIDS (Grimshaw and Fletcher, nd). As combination therapy improves the health of people with HIV/AIDS, demand for social services support is falling and departments may find it difficult to justify specialist HIV teams. As expertise increasingly resides in individuals rather than in departments, Grimshaw and Fletcher feel that employing these people directly may become a preferred option for people with HIV. Current direct payment users with HIV have also suggested that such payments can bring flexibility, more options, continuity, more control and improved health as needs are met more effectively. Of these, flexibility is of particular importance, since the needs of people with HIV can fluctuate from week to week and may not be constant.

Sexuality

For gay men and lesbians, direct payments raise a series of additional issues which have been neglected by the vast majority of commentators. An important contribution comes from a seminar held by BCODP in 1991 to promote the concepts of independent living and personal assistance. In a paper on ‘Independent living, personal assistance, disabled lesbians and disabled gay men’, Killin (1993) sets out some of the practical issues faced by gay and lesbian PA users. Some PAs have been known to be homophobic and have deserted the disabled person once their sexual identity has become known. Particular tension can occur when a PA finds the disabled person sleeping with somebody of the same sex or sees lesbian/gay literature around the house. In some situations, PAs have been known to disclose the sexual orientation of the disabled person to their neighbours, leaving the disabled person vulnerable to verbal or physical abuse. A key issue for many gay/lesbian disabled people is when to disclose their sexuality to their PA – during an initial interview or in casual conversation once employed? (Killin, 1993)

Many of these issues have since been reiterated in PSI/NCIL guidance to local authorities (Hasler et al, 1999, pp 32-3), emphasising the need to consider the complexities of employing PAs for gay men and lesbians. In addition to the risk that the disabled person may be deserted by their PA once their sexuality is known, local authorities need to consider the importance of peer support, maintaining confidentiality and specific measures to consult disabled lesbians and gay men seeking to live independently. Additional issues are also raised by the NCIL's, *The rough guide to managing personal assistants*, which recounts the experiences of male PAs making comments about the women in a gay bar and PAs getting 'chatted up' while they are supposed to be assisting the disabled person (Vasey, 2000). For one direct payment recipient, it is also difficult to stop friends of his PA coming up to socialise with the PA while he is working, since many people on the 'gay scene' already know each other. The same recipient has also experienced situations where PAs have mistakenly assumed that assisting a gay man involves having sex with him and become very interested in knowing all the details of his medical history (Vasey, 2000, pp 20, 81-2).

Ethnicity

Experience of direct payment schemes suggests that making cash payments in lieu of services may be a good way of meeting the needs of people from minority ethnic groups, allowing a precise match of user and worker (Hasler et al, 1999). Despite this, anecdotal evidence is beginning to emerge that people from minority ethnic groups are significantly under-represented and face additional barriers to direct payments (Butt et al, 2000). In Scotland, for example, Witcher et al (2000) found that there were no direct payment recipients at all from minority ethnic communities, while research in the London Borough of Tower Hamlets found that none of the 30 users supported by a local coalition of disabled people were from minority communities (despite the large percentage of minority groups living in the borough) (Maglajlic et al, 2000). Research by the Race Equalities Unit has also suggested that there is a lack of knowledge about direct payments among black disabled people and that this group is often excluded from the planning and implementation of direct payment schemes (Butt and Box, 1997; Bignall and Butt, 2000). In an evaluation of direct payments in Norfolk, all recipients were white, with the exception of one person from Sri Lanka who joined the project at the very end of the evaluation (Dawson, 2000).

In 1998, the Race Equalities Unit and Black Spectrum held a workshop on direct payments for people from minority ethnic groups. With funding from the Rowntree Foundation, key issues from the one-off event were published in the form of a conference report in an attempt to identify and overcome the barriers to direct payments (Butt et al, 2000). Key barriers that prevent people from minority ethnic groups from accessing direct payments were found to include:

- a lack of information, outreach and advice targeted at black and minority ethnic disabled people, their families and communities;
- a lack of support;
- the failure to involve black and minority ethnic people in policy, practice, research and development;
- difficulties in recruiting black and minority ethnic PAs;
- limited knowledge about existing good practice;
- wide variations in policy and practice.

Other debates centred on the role of the family, and participants' views varied considerably. Some delegates suggested that black and Asian people may wish to employ family members as PAs. For others, there was a danger that this would blur the role of family members and reduce the independence of the disabled person. During other presentations, a good practice example was presented from Warwickshire, where the local Council of Disabled People has specific responsibilities for work with black and Asian communities (see Box 37).

In 1999, guidance produced by the PSI and NCIL suggested that 'independent living' can be an alien concept to many cultures, often being interpreted as 'independence from family' (Hasler et al, 1999, pp 29-31). As a result, it may be better to emphasise the overall goals of choice and control. While producing the guidance, work undertaken in a London borough revealed a number of practical lessons about direct payments and people from minority ethnic groups. In particular, the researchers emphasised the need to conduct consultations in

Box 37: Direct payments and ethnicity

The Warwickshire Council of Disabled People has identified a number of key issues concerning direct payments and people from minority ethnic groups:

- The need to recruit black staff
- The importance of role models and peer support
- Supporting family members to understand the concept of independent living
- The need for staff to undergo race and disability training
- The importance of using direct payments to employ black PAs. (quoted in Butt et al, 2000, pp 21-3)

community venues using members of that particular community to carry out the consultation and convey information. Involving community leaders is crucial and all information should be provided in appropriate languages, always being mindful of the linguistic, religious and cultural requirements of different community groups. Although local authorities may agree to employing relatives as PAs if this is the best way of meeting individual need, this may not always be the best option and family support should not be assumed to be a cultural norm (Hasler et al, 1999).

SUMMARY

Direct payments have often been conceptualised from the perspective of people with physical impairments, and there has been little consideration of the additional barriers faced by a variety of other user groups. Although direct payments can have many advantages for disabled parents, people with learning difficulties, people with mental health problems, older people, gay men/lesbians, people with HIV/AIDS and people from minority ethnic communities, these groups have often been excluded from, or found it difficult to access, payment schemes. Although different groups face different obstacles, recurring themes include a lack of appropriate information, a lack of awareness among social workers and a lack of peer support. In many cases, these barriers have been strengthened by the nature of official guidance which insists on direct payment recipients being 'willing and able', fails to recognise the needs of people with mental health problems, prohibits the employment of family members and (initially) excluded older people altogether. While the number of people receiving direct payments is increasing (see Chapter Five), further work will be required to ensure equality of access to payments for all user groups.

SEVEN

The advantages of direct payments

Research to date has highlighted a number of key advantages for recipients of direct payments. These include:

- more responsive services and increased choice and control (Hasler et al, 1999);
- improved morale and mental/psychological wellbeing (Glendinning et al, 2000a);
- a more creative use of resources which may sometimes reduce costs, but which certainly ensures better value for money (Zarb and Nadash, 1994; DoH, 1998c).
- a blurring of the boundary between health and social care (Glendinning et al, 2000a).

Choice and control

It is now widely accepted that direct payments enhance choice and control, and this is often taken for granted without adequately assessing the evidence base. Certainly, all the available research suggests that direct payments are a major step forward, but supporters will need to return to the research findings in order to overcome continuing resistance, constantly making and re-making the case that direct payments enhance choice, control and independence.

In the early 1990s, research into the ILF revealed that making cash payments directly to service users gave a sense of control and choice that could not be achieved via statutory services (see Box 38; Kestenbaum, 1993b; Lakey, 1994). While respondents found directly provided services to be inflexible, costly and severely limited in terms of the availability and level of service on offer, they valued the freedom which ILF payments provided. Receiving money with which to employ their own care assistants enabled them to choose staff with whom they felt at ease and who they felt had the right strengths and skills. The disabled person could also employ someone of a particular sex and select carers who spoke the same language as they did. Above all, however, ILF recipients valued being able to hire staff with whom they felt able to develop a good relationship, choosing people with the right personality to make the care package work.

As a result of this, the disabled people were able to establish and maintain longer lasting relationships with their staff and enjoyed greater continuity of personnel. At the same time, they were also able to create flexible support arrangements to meet often fluctuating needs. Throughout a number of research studies, respondents repeatedly emphasised the control that ILF payments gave

Box 38: Choice and control

For many applicants, the ILF was not just about making up for unavailable statutory services. It was the preferred option. From a disabled person's point of view, the provision of cash makes the important difference between having one's personal life controlled by others and exercising choices and control for oneself. Money has enabled ILF clients not only to avoid going into residential care, but also to determine for themselves the help they require, and how and when they want it to be provided. In many cases, where that freedom and corresponding self-respect are not central components, care in the community may be no better than institutional care. (Kestenbaum, 1993a, p 35)

them and the self-respect that they felt as a result of their status as an employer. Rather than being dependent on others to determine and meet their care needs, the disabled people themselves could determine what Kestenbaum (1993b, p 38) describes as "the what, how, who and when of care arrangements".

In 1993, respondents in Morris' study of disabled people's experiences of community care services emphasised the many advantages which employing PAs could bring:

> "I'm a husband, a father and a breadwinner. And ten years ago I was in an institution where I couldn't even decide when I would go to the toilet."
>
> "It means that I can get up in the morning when I want to, and lead the kind of life that I want to.... To not be reliant on my family and friends ... to keep all that separate [so that] to them I'm me rather than someone who needs help."
>
> "It means exercising choice and control, having the right to choose who gets me up and who puts me to bed."
>
> "I'm living on my own, living in the way I like. I can come and go as I like."
>
> "I employ people ..., which allows me to have the life style that I choose." (Morris, 1993a, pp 125-6)

In 1994, similar findings emerged from Zarb and Nadash's study for the BCODP. For many respondents in this study, indirect/direct payments were crucial in enabling recipients to control the times when support was provided, who was employed, what sort of assistance was provided and how it was provided, thereby enhancing quality of life and personal dignity. Overall, the most important aspect of a payments scheme was found to be having choice and control over one's own support arrangements. This in turn led to more reliable and flexible services that enabled needs to be more fully met:

> "I am in control. I can decide when I want help. The way help is delivered – I feel it is *my* life, not someone else's. You are not fitted in to other people's time table. Freedom – you can choose *who* you have. If you don't like them you can have someone else. You can choose the manner in which a task is performed, unlike when home care staff are used. It releases me to have family as family and friends as friends." (Zarb and Nadash, 1994, p 90; emphasis in the original)

After the implementation of the Community Care (Direct Payments) Act in April 1997, further research has emphasised the centrality of choice and control for direct payment recipients. For Peter Brawley, then chair of Glasgow's Centre for Independent Living, direct payments have been a major step forward for disabled people:

> "For people such as myself, for whom the traditional option would have been institutionalised care, being able to choose a personal assistant has made a great difference. I am living with my wife in the community, going out to work every day. It gives us the chance to maximise our potential and take our proper place in a changed world." (quoted in Hunter, 1999, p 10)

Similar sentiments are echoed by other commentators, who point out that future generations will take direct payments for granted and will not be able to believe that there was ever a time when such payments were not available:

> "The direct payment issue is a prime example of the sort of thing that will astound future generations. It will amaze people to think that there was a time when disabled people were thought unable or untrustworthy to receive, without hesitation, the finance they need for the purchase and organisation of their own assistance." (Mason, quoted in Morris, 1993a, p 164)

In 1999, a study carried out by the Social Services Inspectorate found that direct payments recipients were more satisfied with their care arrangements than people receiving direct services, citing feelings of control as a key factor (Fruin, 2000, pp 15-16). For one service user in particular, a direct payments scheme had "just turned everything around – it has given me self-respect" (quoted in Fruin, 2000, p 16 and DoH/SSI, 1999c, p 19). In Norfolk, all respondents in an evaluation of a local direct payments project saw the scheme as a means of gaining more choice and control in their daily lives, empowering them to live their lives as they chose (Dawson, 2000, p 17). This was also the case in Scotland, where recipients valued the opportunity to exercise choice and control, contrasting this with previous disempowering experiences of direct services:

> "Things couldn't be better now. It's given me much more freedom and control and I play a more active role in family life. Choice, freedom and control sums

> it up for me. It has been amazing, my life has completely changed." (quoted in Witcher et al, 2000, para 6.10)

In Staffordshire, service users also saw direct payments as a means of enhancing their choice, power and control (Leece, 2000), while in Birmingham, direct payments gave recipients greater control over their care arrangements, increasing their independence, quality of life and power over their own situation (Riley, 1999). These were also important issues in a study funded by the Department of Health into direct payments and the health and social care divide (Glendinning et al, 2000a, b, c). By being able to exercise control over the support they received, direct payment recipients were able to tailor care to their individual needs and personal preferences, ensure continuity of care, develop flexible packages of care that encompassed a greater range of tasks and enhance their own independence.

The importance of choice and control has also emerged as a key issue from publications produced by organisations of disabled people such as NCIL. In 1999, PSI/NCIL guidance for local authorities began by stressing that direct payments are a means to an end and a way of achieving independent living:

> Of all the advice given by disabled people who use payment schemes, people who run support schemes for payment users and those who commission payments schemes, one starting point emerges clearly and firmly: it's about independent living. Every aspect of a direct payment system needs to be geared to enabling disabled people to achieve maximum choice and control in their everyday lives. (Hasler et al, 1999, p 5)

A similar message also emerges from NCIL's *The rough guide to managing personal assistants*, which highlights many of the difficulties of employing PAs, but ultimately reiterates the centrality of the increased choice and control that direct payments can bring:

> Disabled people are forever being cast as vulnerable, hence the services that support us tend to be overprotective. Direct Payments are about the right to take risks, to learn, like everyone else does, from our mistakes and to develop into wiser, stronger people. That is independent living.
>
> "Having PAs enabled me to find out who I am and now enables me to be who I am." (Vasey, 2000, pp 129-30)

Morale and wellbeing

For direct payment recipients, feeling in control of their own lives has been found to have important implications for health and wellbeing. There is now a large literature in the field of psychology to suggest that control is essential to wellbeing and is an important element in shaping people's lives and their susceptibility to stress. Often, psychologists distinguish between people who have an internal or an external 'locus of control'. Whereas 'internals' feel in control of what happens to them and that they have the power to influence their lives, 'externals' tend to believe that they have little control over what happens to them since this is the result of outside factors beyond their command (Thompson et al, 1994, pp 54-5). This can be a crucial factor, since research suggests that 'internals' are more successful than 'externals' at work in terms of pay, promotion and job satisfaction, and that they are better able to cope with stress (Andrisani and Nestel, 1976). This has been supported by Kobasa (1979), who suggests that people with a greater sense of control over what happens to them will remain healthier than those who feel powerless in the face of external forces. Another key contribution has been made by Seligman (1975), who believes that 'externals' are more likely to experience 'learned helplessness' (where people who constantly find that they have little power to influence their own destiny lose motivation and give up trying).

With regard to social work, evidence is beginning to emerge that the increased sense of control which receiving direct payments entails can enhance recipients' wellbeing and morale. Certainly, this was one of the key findings to emerge from research into the ILF, which suggested that receiving cash payments enabled some disabled people to remain in the community rather than enter hospital or residential care (Kestenbaum, 1993b). For one service user, Mr R, ILF payments gave him the confidence to do other things, safe in the knowledge that the physical side of his care was under control and that his support arrangements were keeping pressure sores at bay (Kestenbaum, 1993b, p 39). As the government was considering the potential of direct payments in the mid-1990s, moreover, John Evans, the chair of BCODP's Independent Living Committee, was clear that direct payments would have a direct effect on people's quality of life:

> "Direct payments allow disabled people to be less dependent, to have real choices about how we live our lives.... They have a real impact on quality of life – on health, wellbeing, psychological development, and relationships with others." (quoted in George, 1994a, p 14)

After the introduction of direct payments in 1997, research conducted by the PSI/NCIL suggested that replacing directly provided services with cash payments may not only be more cost-efficient, but may also bring a range of additional social and economic benefits:

> Savings may come from a reduction in demand for acute and/or long-term health care on the basis that full independence may well be associated with higher levels of quality of life and the associated benefits in terms of general well-being. (Zarb, 1998, pp 8-9)

Improved mental and physical health was also a key outcome for disabled people during research into direct payments and the health and social care divide (Glendinning et al, 2000a, c). For many direct payment recipients, enhanced choice and control increased their self-confidence, morale and emotional and psychological health in a range of areas. For some respondents, the depth of their relationship with their PA was a crucial source of support and helped to prevent feelings of isolation. For others, the quality of care which they were able to arrange for themselves had a knock-on effect on their attitude to their impairments and symptoms. This was particularly the case for people with mental health problems, who felt that direct payments gave them the confidence and support they needed to recover from their illness. Also during this study, it emerged that some direct payment recipients were using their money to buy health care that had previously been denied to them, receiving valued services which may not otherwise have been available (to be discussed later and in Chapter Eight).

Use of resources

Throughout the implementation of direct payments, issues of cost and of cost-efficiency have been paramount. While the possibility of legislation was being debated in Parliament, government opposition to direct payments was based at least in part on fears about the cost implications of making payments to individuals instead of providing services (see Chapter Three). When direct payments were formally introduced, the accompanying guidance emphasised that:

> A local authority should not make direct payments unless they are at least as cost-effective as the services which it would otherwise arrange. In comparison between the cost of the direct payment and the cost of a service, the local authority should use the full cost of each, taking account of any administrative costs and other overheads. Local authorities may, if they choose, make direct payments at a greater cost than the cost of arranging the equivalent service, provided they are satisfied that this is still at least as cost-effective as arranging services, ie that the increased cost can be justified by the greater effectiveness arising from enabling the person to manage his or her own services and live independently. (DoH, 1997a, p 16)

This was reiterated by the revised 2000 guidance, which added the need to consider long-term best value (DoH, 2000a).

As a result of the recurring emphasis on cost-efficiency, much of the research to date on direct payments has included a consideration of financial matters and value for money. In many cases, this has even happened in studies where the researchers do not appear to value cost-efficiency themselves, but feel the need to include a discussion of this issue because of its centrality to the government's agenda. For this reason, there is a substantial body of literature that suggests that direct payments are much more cost-effective than directly provided services and, in some studies, may sometimes even be cheaper than traditional services as well.

Certainly, this has been the case with the ILF, which has been found to be around 30% cheaper than direct services (quoted in Mandelstam, 1999, p 233). Prior to the implementation of direct payments, moreover, Morris wrote that "enabling people to employ their own personal assistants is a more cost-effective way of meeting personal assistance needs than using local authority home care services" (Morris, 1993a, p 168). This assertion appeared to be based primarily on research conducted as part of an evaluation of the Personal Assistance Advisor post at Greenwich Association of Disabled People (Oliver and Zarb, 1992). Even when the cost of the support provided by the advisor was taken into account, the scheme still appeared to be cheaper than providing services directly. As Conservative Minister, Nicholas Scott, wrote in his foreword to the evaluation:

> This report on Personal Assistance Schemes in Greenwich shows that as well as being cost effective, such schemes offer disabled people a greater degree of independence when compared with traditional forms of provision. (Oliver and Zarb, 1992)

Perhaps the most influential study of all was carried out by Zarb and Nadash (1994) on behalf of the BCODP, specifically seeking to address issues of cost-efficiency in response to the then Conservative government's reluctance to legalise direct payments (see also Evans and Hasler, 1996). In order to compare the care packages of service users receiving some form of payment with those of people receiving direct services, the study sought to calculate unit costs for both types of support, taking account of all the expenditure involved. This included the direct costs and overheads associated with traditional services, as well as the direct and indirect costs of using payments to purchase care directly (for example, wages, recruitment and management costs and incidental costs such as support workers' travel expenses). Although the methodology for compiling and comparing this data was complex, the researchers concluded that care packages financed by direct/indirect payments were, on average, some 30% to 40% cheaper than directly provided services (see Table 10). In addition to this, the researchers also noted that the concept of 'cost-efficiency' should incorporate not only issues of cost, but also a consideration of quality. That direct payments resulted in higher quality services had already been demonstrated earlier in the study, where payment recipients suggested that:

- payment schemes met a wider range of needs than traditional services and led to fewer unmet needs;
- people receiving payments have more reliable support and experience fewer problems with their care;
- payment recipients express higher levels of satisfaction than people using directly provided services. (Zarb and Nadash, 1994, pp 142-3)

Table 10: Average hourly unit costs

Type of care package	Average hourly unit costs of care
Direct/indirect payments	£5.18
Directly provided services	£8.52

Source: Zarb and Nadash (1994, pp 117-43)

Overall, therefore, the researchers were adamant that making payments to disabled service users was extremely cost-effective, not only representing a cheaper option than directly provided services, but also achieving better results for service users (see also Table 10 and Box 39):

> In other words, every pound spent through a payments scheme not only goes further than a pound spent on services, but also purchases assistance of a higher quality. According to the definition of cost-efficiency outlined above, therefore, direct/indirect payments clearly represent better value for money than direct service provision. (Zarb and Nadash, 1994, p 143)

After the implementation of direct payments, research has continued to emphasise the cost-efficiency of paying money directly to disabled people. In West Sussex, a new direct payments scheme was reported to have made direct savings of £30,000 per year for just 15 recipients, while at the same time enabling them to purchase additional hours of care that would have cost £23,000 if delivered by in-house services (quoted in Hasler, 1999, p 7). In Scotland, research suggests that direct payments can lead to a more efficient use of human and financial

Box 39: Costs and benefits of direct payments

What the research evidence tells us is that direct payments have consistently been shown to be a cost effective mechanism for enabling disabled people to access high quality support which maximises choice and control at equivalent or, often, lower cost than other forms of community based support. The most detailed study carried out in the UK, for example, showed that support packages based on direct payments were on average 30 to 40 per cent cheaper than equivalent directly provided services. This study also highlighted very clearly that people receiving direct or indirect payments had higher overall levels of satisfaction with their support arrangements than service users. This was particularly noticeable in relation to reliability and flexibility and the degree of confidence people had in their support arrangements being able to meet their needs.

Other smaller scale studies have shown similar results. The evidence from this research demonstrates that user controlled money goes further, so investing in independent living is a more cost-effective use of public finance. (Zarb, 1998, p 1)

resources, while also improving the quality and appropriateness of care (Witcher et al, 2000, para 7.8). In particular, the researchers found that time invested in setting up direct payments schemes can be recouped in the medium/long-term, that direct payments can be cheaper than using agency care and that direct payments improve quality by enabling needs to be met more effectively. In Norfolk, it proved difficult to calculate some of the hidden costs associated with a direct payments scheme (see Chapter Eight), but an evaluation still concluded that direct payments were a more cost-effective option than traditional services. This was despite the fact that the support arrangements in this particular scheme were extremely complex and that responsibility was split between two different agencies, thus duplicating a number of costs:

> Direct payments are a cheaper alternative than direct service provision or contracted agency service and become cheaper still comparatively over time. The present scheme could become more cost effective by using one support agency rather than two.... It is difficult to envisage an alternative means of delivering a community care service ... which would be cheaper than a direct payments scheme. (Dawson, 2000, p 46)

Elsewhere, anecdotal evidence suggests that direct payments may not necessarily be cheaper than directly provided services, but certainly represent value for money. This is the opinion expressed by Roy Taylor, Director of Community Services for the Royal Borough of Kingston-upon-Thames and a former chair of the ADSS Disabilities Committee. In a Department of Health (1998c) promotional video, Taylor warns against the assumption that direct payments will necessarily result in huge savings for local authorities, but does emphasise that:

- disabled people have shown themselves to be very innovative and creative in designing care packages for themselves;
- disabled people are in control of their payments and want to use this money as effectively as possible;
- often disabled people can make better use of their payments than the local authority could.

The health and social care divide

In Britain, health and social services have traditionally fallen under the remit of two separate agencies. During the postwar welfare reforms of the 1940s, two separate pieces of legislation established a fundamental and enduring distinction between health care (for the sick) and social care (for people in need of care and attention), which continues to dominate service provision to this day. Described by the New Labour government in terms of a "Berlin Wall" (HCD, 09/12/1997, col 802), the health and social care divide has frequently been identified as a major source of confusion and complexity for service users and patients, leading to fragmented care and uncertainty about which agency is responsible for which service (see for example, Henwood and Wistow, 1993; Royal Commission on Long-Term Care, 1999; Glasby and Littlechild, 2000b; Hudson, 2000; Twigg, 2000). Through a number of research studies, key divisions between health and social services have been shown to include:

- structural fragmentation and complexity;
- procedural differences;
- financial differences;
- professional differences;
- differences in status and legitimacy (Hudson, 2000, p 254).

For frontline practitioners and individual service users alike, these divisions have serious consequences, making an already difficult job much harder and potentially culminating in a breakdown in people's care arrangements (see Box 40). Despite attempts to achieve a "seamless service" in which health and social care is experienced by service users and patients as a continuity (DoH/SSI, 1991), the government has not yet been able to resolve the issues raised by the health and social care divide, and success remains as elusive as ever (Glasby, 2000a, b, 2001b; Glasby and Littlechild, 2000b, c).

Against this background, direct payments have been found to have the potential to provide greater continuity for disabled people and to be able to begin to overcome the artificial divisions which the health and social care divide engenders. Although policy and practice guidance forbids the provision of payments by the health service or to purchase health care (DoH, 1997a), it is possible for health authorities to transfer funds under section 28 of the 1977 NHS Act to contribute to direct payments packages (Glendinning et al, 2000b). While the blurring of the boundaries between health and social care can have disadvantages as well as advantages (see Chapter Eight), it does appear to enable disabled people to take greater control of their lives and construct care packages in a way that genuinely meets their needs. To date, this is particularly apparent

Box 40: The health and social care divide

For front-line workers, the need to overcome a tangle of legal, administrative and organisational obstacles in order to work effectively across service boundaries with colleagues from other professions and backgrounds is an almost daily struggle. Whether it is hospital discharge, continuing care, domiciliary care in the community or rehabilitation, the boundaries between these services are an almost constant source of difficulty, debate and consternation. For individual service users who find themselves trapped between these two large and powerful agencies, the experience is frequently one of frustration, disillusionment and despair. In extreme cases, it is not unknown for a patient to fail to meet the criteria for either health or social care, falling between the boundaries of existing service provision and being passed backwards and forwards until a major crisis occurs. (Glasby and Littlechild, 2000b, p 4) in three main studies (Hasler et al, 1999; Kestenbaum, 1999; Glendinning et al, 2000a, b, c), all of which took place in the late 1990s as the New Labour government was seeking to grapple with the issue of joint working across the health and social care divide (see, for example, DoH, 1998a, d, 2000d, e).

In research funded by the Joseph Rowntree Foundation, Kestenbaum (1999) found that people with high support needs had very different outcomes depending on how well their local and health authorities were able to work together. While people in one area were able to benefit from a multi-disciplinary Community Multiple Sclerosis Team, other respondents found it difficult to get a contribution from the NHS towards their care packages or could become involved in demarcation disputes between health and social service providers. Despite this, there were some positive examples of disabled people receiving payments which had been funded by both health and social services, and Kestenbaum (1999, p 49) concluded that "the introduction of direct payments in particular can successfully challenge current rigidities [between health and social care]." For many service users, physiotherapy was a particular priority and an area where PAs could be trained to provide support. In one specific example, a disabled person (Dan) had a weekly care package costing over £900, funded by a combination of his own income, local authority contributions, health authority contributions and ILF payments (p 47). As part of this package, it was agreed that a community physiotherapist would train Dan's care workers to provide regular physiotherapy.

Also in 1999, the PSI and NCIL published guidance for local authorities based on research into the implementation of direct payments (Hasler et al, 1999). In a one-page chapter focusing on health and continuing care issues, the guidance emphasises that it may be more cost-effective for health authorities to transfer money to local authorities in cases where the disabled person is using direct payments to employ a PA. This is particularly the case when the disabled person needs physiotherapy or help with catheter/ventilator care, since the PA can be trained to do these tasks and prevent the need for nursing input. If these arrangements are to be successful, however, training issues will need to be addressed and there may need to be formal protocols for establishing how much money will be provided by the health authority. One method of clarifying these issues is for local authorities to formalise their relationship with their health colleagues through the local continuing care agreement.

In 2000, research funded by the Department of Health and carried out by the National Primary Care Research and Development Centre focused on direct payments and the boundaries between health and social care (Glendinning et al, 2000a). Through interviews and focus groups with direct payment recipients, PAs and health and social care professionals, the study found that few disabled people made a distinction between health and social care, using terms such as 'personal care' to refer to their support needs:

> "In my mind you can't split personal care into separate compartments – personal care, health care, social care. It's a holistic approach, it's the well-being of the whole person. Every part of care, whether it's domestic or ... it

> all contributes to the well-being and health of the whole person." (Glendinning et al, 2000c, p 12)

In particular, respondents adopted four approaches when arguing against the principle of separate categories of health and social care:

- Disabled people need a holistic approach that supersedes notions of health and social care (see above quote).
- Social care needs only arise because of underlying health problems.
- Social care reduces the risk of health problems.
- Social care contributes to greater wellbeing and therefore to emotional and mental health.

During the study, it became apparent that many participants were using direct payments to purchase care that would traditionally be defined as health care (such as physiotherapy, assistance with medication, and bladder and bowel management). This was felt by the disabled people concerned to compensate for shortages in existing health services and to provide greater choice, control and independence. As a result, many respondents wanted direct payments to be extended to cover a wider range of health care (such as chiropody, physiotherapy and nursing care), to clarify exactly whether they should be spending their payments on such services and to be able to purchase health-related equipment (such as continence supplies or wheelchairs). Despite this, the use of direct payments to finance health care could also be problematic, raising a range of issues concerning training, supervision, risk and equity (see Chapter Eight). While major reservations remain, the researchers' overall conclusion was that:

> The current organisational, budgetary and professional divisions between 'health' and 'social' services still apparently fail to recognise and respond appropriately to [the] realities of disabled people's lives. (Glendinning et al, 2000b, p 199)

> It is clear that direct payments can ... help disabled people to construct their own integrated services which breach the 'Berlin Wall' between health and social services to a limited extent and that there is potential for this to be extended. (Glendinning et al, 2000a, p 47)

SUMMARY

Although they bring a range of advantages for disabled people, it is important to return to evidence from research in order to overcome continued opposition to direct payments. To date, research into the ILF, indirect payments and direct payments suggests that replacing directly provided services with some sort of payment scheme can enhance choice and control, improve health and wellbeing and begin to blur the traditional and artificial boundaries between health and social care. While opinion is divided as to whether or not direct payments are actually cheaper than providing services directly, there is some evidence that this may be the case. In any event, direct payments are certainly more cost-effective, improving continuity, satisfaction and flexibility and enabling disabled people to commission care that genuinely meets their needs.

EIGHT

Possible difficulties

As the previous chapter has demonstrated, direct payments bring a range of tangible benefits which can enhance the choice, control and wellbeing of recipients. We have also seen how pressure for direct payments built up over a long period (Chapters Two to Five) and how organisations of disabled people were able to mount a sustained campaign for the new legislation to be introduced. As a result of this, direct payments are almost always viewed as an essentially positive policy measure, and have probably been subjected to less careful analysis and critical reflection than should perhaps be the case. While direct payments *do* bring a number of very real advantages for service users, there are a number of limitations and contradictions that workers and service users need to consider:

- Are direct payments the product of a government seeking to restrict public spending and introduce a flawed notion of consumerism into community care services?
- Could direct payments represent a subtle shift in the boundary between health and social care?
- Does the success of direct payments rely too heavily on the attitudes and training of frontline workers?
- Are direct payments schemes adequately financed and do recipients receive enough money to purchase sufficient care?
- Might direct payments lead to the greater exploitation of women?
- Could direct payments leave service users vulnerable to abuse or at risk of significant harm?
- Is there a risk that some authorities could use direct payments to distance themselves from service users they perceive as 'troublemakers'?
- Are the practicalities of managing direct payments prohibitive?

Consumerism and public expenditure

Although direct payments offer a range of social service users increased choice and control (see Chapter Seven), it is often forgotten that the 1996 Community Care (Direct Payments) Act was introduced by a Conservative government firmly committed to New Right or neo-liberal social and economic policies. Building on the work of thinkers such as Hayek (1944), Friedman (1962) and, more recently, Murray (1984), the New Right approach has been summarised in terms of a belief in three key issues:

- the free market;
- the minimal state;
- individual liberty and responsibility. (Adams, 1998, p 85)

Within social policy, this has led to a neo-liberal critique of state welfare which acquired increasing significance after the economic crises and political polarisation of the 1970s. As Alcock explains:

> [The New Right's] main argument was that state intervention to provide welfare services ... merely drove up the cost of public expenditure to a point where it began to interfere with the effective operation of a market economy. They claimed that this was a point that had already been reached in Britain in the 1970s as the high levels of taxation needed for welfare services had reduced profits, crippled investment and driven capital overseas. [At the same time] the New Right also challenged the desirability of state welfare in practice, arguing that free welfare services only encouraged feckless people to become dependent upon them and provided no incentive for individuals and families to protect themselves through savings or insurance. Furthermore, right-wing theorists claimed that state monopoly over welfare services reduced the choices available to people to meet their needs in a variety of ways and merely perpetuated professionalism and bureaucracy. (1996, p 12)

After the election of Margaret Thatcher as Prime Minister in 1979, these ideas acquired increasing support at the heart of central government, culminating in a series of market-led reforms in traditional public sector services such as education, housing and the NHS. Within community care, such reforms were to transform social services departments from direct service providers into service purchasers, with an explicit brief to purchase a significant amount of care from the independent sector (Lewis, 1996). These changes were presented as "promoting choice and independence" and giving "people a greater individual say in how they live their lives and the services they need to help them do so" (DoH, 1989, p 4). This has been described by Means and Smith as promoting a form of "empowerment by exit":

> 'Exit' is essentially a market approach which seeks to empower consumers by giving them a choice between alternatives and the option of 'exit' from a service and/or provider, if dissatisfied. The consumer, in other words, will be able to change provider, and if a large number of them make the same decision about the same provider then that provider will be punished for their inefficiency by going out of 'business'. (1998a, p 83)

Although neo-liberal attempts to recast service users as consumers have undoubtedly led to greater emphasis on service quality and on meeting individual needs, a consumerist approach to social policy has been criticised by a number of commentators (see, for example, Barnes and Walker, 1996; Means and Smith, 1998a). As Marian Barnes has suggested, empowerment by exit and the consumerist philosophy on which this is based both rely on a number of essential preconditions:

- Alternatives need to exist.
- The person concerned needs access to information not only about alternatives, but also about characteristics of alternatives which might suggest that they would overcome dissatisfaction with existing services, but also not substitute new for existing problems.
- Moving from one option to another should be practically possible.
- Moving from one option to another should not of itself generate damaging disruption. (1997, p 34)

As Barnes continues: "If one considers the circumstances in which most people use health and social care services, it is clear that all these circumstances will rarely apply".

In addition to promoting the notion of welfare recipients as consumers, the New Right has also emphasised the need to curtail public spending on welfare. As we have seen in Chapter Two, the ILF introduced in 1988 was restricted in 1993 as a result of concerns about the rapidly increasing cost of such schemes. We have also seen in Chapters Three and Four how financial concerns thwarted previous attempts to introduce direct payments in the early 1990s and how government guidance emphasised the need for direct payments to be at least as cost-effective as the services that they replace. Although the 1996 Community Care (Direct Payments) Act was introduced three years after the reform of the ILF, this was seen as less of a financial threat to the government since direct payments were to be operated by local authorities within their existing cash-limited budgets (Means and Smith, 1998a, p 85).

Against this background, the introduction of direct payments begins to take on a new and slightly more sinister appearance. While direct payments undoubtedly bring a number of very real benefits to service users, it is also possible to see the 1996 Act as an attempt by government to promote a discredited and flawed notion of 'empowerment by exit' and to do so in a way that would not result in an escalation of public expenditure. In such a scenario, it would be left to local authority social services departments to balance the books and reconcile the very real demand for direct payments with already stringent budget constraints (Glasby and Glasby, 1999). While this should not prevent service users from benefiting from the many advantages of direct payments, it does suggest that there may be conflicting agendas surrounding direct payments, with service users and central government each wanting different things from the reforms. This contradiction has been identified most forcefully by Pearson (2000), who emphasises the tensions between the social justice discourse of the disability movement and the market discourse of government. For frontline workers, such tensions may ultimately lead to role conflict as they try to support direct payment recipients, while at the same time working within a system and within financial constraints that are not always as emancipatory as the initial concept of direct payments may suggest.

The health and social care divide

Under the 1996 Community Care (Direct Payments) Act, social services departments may only make payments to service users in lieu of community care services and these funds cannot be used to purchase health care:

> Direct payments will only be available in lieu of community care services which would otherwise have been arranged by the local authority. Direct payments will *not* replace care provided by the NHS. (DoH/Scottish Office/Welsh Office/Northern Ireland Office, 1996; emphasis in the original)
>
> The Act *does not* authorise any other body, such as a health authority or a housing authority, to make direct payments; nor does it enable direct payments to be used to purchase health or housing services. (DoH, 1997a, p 3; emphasis in the original)

Despite this, evidence is beginning to emerge that direct payment recipients may be using their money to purchase tasks that would traditionally be seen as the responsibility of the NHS, blurring the often problematic boundary between health and social care. In the late 1990s, the Department of Health commissioned the National Primary Care Research and Development Centre to undertake a programme of research on the boundaries between these two services. One study focused on direct payments, identifying three case study direct payment schemes and carrying out semi-structured in-depth interviews with 42 direct payment users and 13 health professionals, telephone interviews with seven health and local authority managers, and focus groups with 14 PAs (Glendinning et al, 2000a).

As noted in Chapter Seven, the distinction between health and social care often has little relevance from the perspective of the service user and can frequently cause a range of practical and administrative difficulties for workers seeking to support people with complex needs (Glasby and Littlechild, 2000b). To overcome some of these difficulties, some direct payments recipients in the Glendinning study used their money to purchase support with tasks such as administering medication, physiotherapy exercises, bladder/bowel management, changing dressings and aromatherapy treatments – all areas which might be seen as falling under the remit of the NHS. While some people had decided to use direct payments in this way as a result of the greater choice and independence which direct payments offered, the most common reason was the shortage of mainstream health services (see Box 41). In particular, some participants had experienced restrictions on physiotherapy input and funding/staffing shortages in community nursing and rehabilitation services, using their direct payments to compensate for these shortfalls. In other cases, there was a clear sense that NHS services can be deliberately withdrawn once it becomes apparent that a PA is being employed by the disabled person. Often, this was something that was not openly discussed and that did not lead to health authority input into direct payment packages. As a result, it seems as though some disabled people may

Box 41: NHS withdrawal?

"Once you've turned 16, generally speaking the health service doesn't give a toss about you. You're not followed up, you're not getting anything regular, until something serious has gone wrong with you."

"To be honest the district nurses were putting verbal pressures on me that they are health carers not social carers and they did want to move away from doing that kind of work, it was obvious that was what they wanted."

"[District nurses] don't do any of that now, it's all done by personal assistants. Once they see that our personal assistants are capable of doing it, they pass it on."

"If you're severely disabled, you're going to need long-term physio. Why should it come out of social services' budget when it's a health thing? Often they try to dump their costs on social services." (Glenndinning et al, 2000a, p 14)

effectively be forced into using money paid to them by social services for social care needs in order to meet their health care needs. For the researchers, this represented "a de facto transfer of responsibility for the cost of healthcare from the NHS to local authority social services authorities" and a "a hidden shift across the 'health'/'social' care divide" (Glendinning et al, 2000a, pp 14, 42).

The National Primary Care Research and Development Centre study not only raises issues about the boundary between health and social care, but also has significant implications for training, supervision and health and safety. Some direct payment recipients were worried that their PAs would not have access to the training and support that they would need in order to carry out further 'health' tasks. Should this training be available, however, it may ultimately turn user-controlled PAs into more autonomous semi-professionals, replicating the limitations of directly provided services, disempowering service users and undermining the fundamental tenets of direct payments. For some PAs, there was reluctance to take on some health care tasks and concerns that PAs had little formal guidance about the tasks they should be performing, negotiating their role directly with the disabled person. Some felt they had insufficient training to take on particular tasks and were angry on their employers' behalf about the withdrawal of health services. Others were concerned about the risks of infection while performing invasive procedures or of injury to their employer while undertaking physiotherapy exercises. Overall, there was a clear consensus that greater training was required in basic skills such as resuscitation, lifting and handling and food preparation; while some people suggested that additional specialist training should be provided by the NHS in basic physiotherapy, changing catheters, applying dressings and administering injections.

Among frontline practitioners and their managers, there was an awareness that PAs were carrying out health care tasks for recipients of direct payments and concerns about what would happen if health professionals became more involved in training and supervising PAs. Some workers were anxious about the resources and expertise that would be required to train PAs, while others felt that they would need to exercise considerable control over PAs if they were to become responsible for the quality of their work. Clearly, the latter view is somewhat at odds with the original concept of direct payments as a means of enhancing the control of disabled people over their own lives and services. Extending the health role of PAs was also felt to raise issues concerning the fragmentation of services between various carers, a potential loss of control by statutory agencies and who would have access to confidential information about the disabled person's medical condition. For disabled people, PAs, practitioners and managers alike there was anxiety that using direct payments to fund health care could challenge the principles of the NHS and create a two-tier system in which some disabled people are able to purchase better health care than non-recipients of direct payments.

While the National Primary Care Research and Development Centre research is very much an exploratory study into a previously unresearched area, it does raise fundamental issues for the future concerning the health and social care divide and the unforeseen impact that direct payments may have on access to health care.

The 'gatekeeping' role of social workers

Time and time again, a major barrier to an extension of direct payments has been shown to be the anxiety and ignorance of frontline social workers. This was widely anticipated as the 1996 Act was being implemented (Oliver and Sapey, 1999), and subsequent events have tended to support those uncertain about the capacity of social services departments to embrace the significant changes implied by the direct payments legislation. In Scotland, for example, practitioners were deterred by perceived expenditure and workload implications, by a lack of understanding of direct payments, or by a fear of a loss of control (Witcher et al, 2000). Others feared that service users would misspend their payments on drugs or alcohol and there was a widespread suggestion that senior managers may be deliberately 'blocking' the implementation of the 1996 legislation. Overall, understanding of direct payments was limited, with some departments unsure of the differences between direct and indirect payments.

Elsewhere (Fruin, 2000, p 17), the Social Services Inspectorate has found evidence of an ambivalent attitude to direct payments among staff:

> "I am very worried about direct payments – vulnerable people managing their own services." (social worker in a multi-disciplinary team)

> "Can I risk [direct payments] ... on behalf of clients?" (adults team social worker)

Some members of staff lacked knowledge about direct payments legislation and about local procedures, disadvantaging their service users. In the local inspections, direct payments sometimes had a low profile among non-specialist workers and might not be adequately publicised through fears that this would create additional demands on already stretched budgets. On one occasion, proposals for a direct payments scheme were hindered by the lack of a champion to drive forward the project and a lack of understanding about the role that direct payments could play in the range of services designed to support independent living (DoH/SSI, 1999a, b, c). Similar findings were also to emerge from Norfolk (Dawson, 2000) and Staffordshire, where an evaluation of a direct payments pilot project emphasised the need to promote awareness of direct payments not only among disabled people, but also among social workers (Leece, 2000, pp 39-40).

In West Sussex, social workers were found to have very little knowledge of direct payments, with some practitioners claiming that people with learning difficulties could not receive direct payments but that disabled children could (quoted in Leece, 2000, p 39). Findings such as these supported previous research in London, which suggested that people at all levels – users, carers and junior members of staff – have little knowledge of direct payments (Brandon et al, 2000; Maglajlic et al, 2000). In the case of people with learning difficulties, interviews with 10 users, 10 carers and 10 members of staff found that only two members of staff out of the 30 people interviewed had even heard of direct payments (Maglajlic et al, 2000, pp 100-1). For older people, research carried out by Age Concern suggests that few staff within social services knew anything about direct payments (even in areas with a history of them), raising serious questions as to how service users were to be kept informed (Age Concern, 1998; see also Box 42).

Elsewhere, it may not just be ignorance or lack of training which hinders the implementation and take-up of direct payments, but political and/or professional opposition. Depending on the political views of local councillors and social services managers, some authorities may view direct payments as a threat to their own in-house domiciliary and day care (George, 1996), representing a form of "privatisation by the back door" (Hasler et al, 1999, p 7). At the same time, direct payments might be expected to lead to a change in social work practice, prompting a shift away from providing/purchasing services *for* disabled people to supporting them to purchase their own care. This feature of direct payments is particularly identified by Dawson (2000) in her evaluation of the Norfolk Independent Living Project. During the study, it became apparent that a significant majority of people without previous experience of indirect payment schemes heard of direct payments through their social worker, but that some practitioners were withholding this information. Whereas staff specialising in work with people with physical impairments were familiar with the concept of indirect payments, workers from mental health or learning difficulty teams had little knowledge of users purchasing their own care. As the evaluation progressed, it became clear that the introduction of direct payments involved "a change of culture" within the social services department, in which

Box 42: Lack of information

"The information that gets here is lousy. Sometimes they tell you something, like 'you can have this'.... And then they say that it's going to be in two months, three months ... and then you hear nothing else about it." (Maglajlic et al, 2000, p 101)

"My social worker had difficulty accessing relevant information. Her manager did not have the answers to her questions and could not tell her where to find the answer." (Leece, 2000, p 39)

Despite widespread information campaigns, many people with learning difficulties still know nothing about direct payments. (Bewley, 2000a, p 14)

As the Direct Payments pilot project progressed, it became increasingly apparent that the single most significant factor in determining who became an employer through direct payments was the potential employer's social worker. (Dawson, 2000, p 22)

Amanda Anderson (not her real name) ... believes that social workers are not properly trained to help disabled people with direct payments. Her social worker put together a 'completely unworkable' care plan timed to the last minute, she says.... "She had allowed two minutes each day for whoever helped me to put my bag in the car. But most days something happens that isn't on the time plan, say, my cat is sick on the carpet. While my assistant is clearing that up she has missed three jobs according to the care plan!" Anderson is still negotiating improvements in the rigid timetable with her social worker. (Valois, 2000b, p 21)

individual social workers were having to take on more of an enabling role (Dawson, 2000, p 53). While some workers relished this role, others may have been less enthusiastic, and the take-up of direct payments was directly linked to the approach of individual workers (see also Box 43).

In many ways, the crucial role of social workers in encouraging or preventing disabled people from accessing direct payments is hardly surprising. Previous research into the information provided by social services departments has suggested that inefficient distribution systems and poor targeting can prevent information from reaching the right people at the right time and in the right place. Although many authorities produce material in different formats and languages, most information is in standard print (Fryer, 1998). Even where authorities make considerable efforts to produce accessible information for minority groups, the publicity and leaflets that do exist may not always find their way to the people who need them (DoH/SSI, 1997). For disabled people trying to make sense of the complexities of social services bureaucracy, the difficulty of obtaining accessible information about the options open to them has been well documented (see Box 44 and Beardshaw, 1988; Zarb and Oliver, 1993; Barnes, 1995; Davis et al, 1997 and so on). In one research project, two case study social services departments were not providing disabled people with

Box 43: The role of care management

My involvement in the promotion of direct payments does raise questions for me about the current state of play in care management. Care managers are extremely important gatekeepers in the whole direct payments story. I have a strong impression that people with learning difficulties who have been able to access direct payments have always had a champion on their side. This has often been a forward-thinking (and tenacious) family member, independent advisor, advocate or, sometimes, care manager. These care managers have been vital in the promotion of direct payments so far but they are not the majority within social services. If direct payments are to become an easy mainstream option ... then enabling people to access them must become normal care management practice. For this to happen, significant change is required to individual, team and organisational practice around care management.... The care management system is under many pressures and the truth is that direct payments are not a daily priority for many care managers.... This is a shame because the ethos of direct payments is extremely exciting. Care managers now have the chance to actually give service users the money to buy their own services. This sharing of power, this chance to see individual lives flourish whilst practical support needs are met, is a fantastic opportunity for care managers to be inspired by their job. The opportunity is there. (Bewley, 2000a, pp 14-15)

the information and advice they needed, since frontline staff saw requests for information as potential demands on their services (Davis et al, 1997). Elsewhere, the Social Services Inspectorate has found that information for disabled people may be out of date and repetitive, not specific to disabled people, inaccessible to people from minority ethnic groups and poorly distributed (DoH/SSI, 1996).

At the same time, it has long been recognised that social workers occupy a crucial gatekeeping role and can work in a number of informal ways to limit the demands made upon them (Rees, 1978; Satyamurti, 1981). Described by Lipsky (1980) as "street level bureaucrats", social workers have been shown to use their professional discretion in order to balance competing priorities and to protect themselves against the overwhelming pressures that they face (see Box 45). Often, they will seek to manage their workloads by making assumptions about their service users, categorising them and forming stereotypical responses

Box 44: Access to information

Information is also a key pre-requisite to disabled people having genuine choice and control over how their needs are to be met. Without information about available resources, how to access services, or about their rights, it is impossible for people to make genuine choices or determine what kind of support is most appropriate to meet their self-defined needs. However, previous research has often highlighted information poverty as a major constraint on providing appropriate and adequate solutions to disabled people's support needs. (Zarb and Oliver, 1993, p 9)

Box 45: Street-level bureaucracy

The decisions of street-level bureaucrats, the routines they establish, and the devices they invent to cope with uncertainties and work pressures, effectively become the public policies they carry out.... Public policy is not best understood as made in legislatures or top-floor suites of high-ranking administrators, because in important ways it is actually made in the crowded offices and daily encounters of street-level workers. (Lipsky, 1980, p xii)

to their needs, thereby adding a degree of stability and predictability to their work. Although the concept of street-level bureaucracy was initially applied to the reorganisation of social services departments in the 1970s, research funded by the Joseph Rowntree Foundation has demonstrated that frontline practitioners continue to behave in similar ways (Davis et al, 1997; Ellis et al, 1999). Based on observations of social work assessments and interviews with users and carers, the study found that workers used screening mechanisms, computer-based assessments and eligibility criteria to manage demand, thereby rationing their time and resources. Although the methods of rationing would appear to have changed since the 1970s, the gatekeeping role of social workers is just as real.

Against this background, the success of direct payments is likely to continue to be closely linked to the attitudes and actions of frontline staff, and it will be important to ensure that practitioners receive sufficient information and training to be able to become forces for change rather than obstacles to progress (see Chapter Ten).

Financial difficulties

The financial implications of making cash payments to disabled people are an issue that has continued to be debated throughout the campaign for direct payments and the subsequent implementation and expansion of the 1996 Act. Although there is clear evidence that direct payments are a more cost-effective option than directly provided services, this may be because cash payments are likely to lead to more creative care packages that really meet the needs of recipients, and not necessarily because they are actually cheaper (Chapter Seven). We have also already seen how the motives of central government may be influenced by a neo-liberal belief in rolling back the welfare state (as discussed previously) and how concerns about public expenditure thwarted a series of early attempts to legalise direct payments in the early 1990s (Chapter Three). Against this background, there is a growing consensus that financial concerns may be a major obstacle to the success and progress of direct payments, preventing some local authorities from promoting their schemes and potentially leaving recipients with insufficient funds to purchase adequate care.

As noted in Chapter Five, a key barrier to the implementation of direct payments has been a lack of pump-priming to establish schemes with an appropriate support infrastructure (Wellard, 1999). Direct payments may be more cost-effective than direct services when a successful scheme is up and running, but there are workload and cost implications in seeking to set up such a scheme in the first place. In Oxfordshire, for example, the Social Services Inspectorate found that the need to make budget reductions of £10 million over three years impacted significantly on its services for disabled people (DoH/SSI, 1999d). In light of its financial difficulties, Oxfordshire social services department decided that it would be too expensive to establish and support a direct payments scheme with a large infrastructure (such as a centre for independent living), opting instead for a much smaller advice service. In Scotland, research has found that lack of resources can be a major barrier and that some workers can be discouraged by significant increases in their workload as schemes are in their infancy and in areas where support mechanisms for direct payment users are limited (Witcher et al, 2000). In many cases, direct schemes were financed from generic community care budgets, with no additional funding. For departments already struggling to manage over-stretched budgets (Glasby and Glasby, 1999), this can presumably prove a major disincentive to promoting direct payments as an option for disabled people. As one director of social services commented: "There won't be any extra provision in the revenue support grant, and direct payments could in fact attract more people into community care and so create additional demand. This could lead to delays in community care assessments, which are already a problem in many places" (quoted in George, 1996, p 24). Unfortunately, this was an issue that was identified as a potential problem from the very beginning, but one which is still to be adequately addressed:

> Funding could also prove to be a problem.... The pump priming and on-going revenue we have asked for shows little sign of materialising. This is an issue on which we will need to pitch hard for during the expenditure round.... If the goal is to extend basic direct payments schemes on a widespread basis then pump priming will be necessary. If pressure for an even greater coverage becomes intense, then significant additional funds may be needed. (Taylor, 1996c, pp 9-10)

Elsewhere, there was evidence of considerable financial implications in an evaluation carried out in Norfolk (Dawson, 2000). Although direct payment packages were found to be cheaper than directly provided services, this comparison did not take account of a number of 'hidden costs' during the early stages of the direct payments scheme. In this particular case study, implementing direct payments required management time, a seconded worker to reassess people transferring from a previous third-party scheme and a range of consultative and team meetings (see Box 46). Negotiations were also extremely complex, requiring a commitment from senior management and considerable partnership working with a range of disability groups. Although the majority of these start-up costs were incurred early on in the scheme and may be expected to decrease as direct payments become more firmly established,

Box 46: Hidden costs

Cost of direct payments, 1999-2000:	£735,867
Estimated cost of equivalent services:	£764,560
Hidden costs:	Management time A seconded worker Consultation Team meetings Negotiating and setting up support services Establishing system for monitoring and payment

(Adapted from Dawson, 2000, pp 43-4)

the investment required to implement a direct payments scheme does have financial implications which may concern some local authorities.

If financial concerns can create difficulties for local authorities, they can also be extremely detrimental to recipients of direct payments. Prior to the implementation of direct payments, Morris' (1993a) study of community care services for disabled people revealed how indirect payment schemes and ILF contributions often failed to take account of indirect costs. These included extra expenditure on food, entertainment and transport when being accompanied by a PA, as well as the costs of being an employer (for example, National Insurance contributions, liability insurance, recruitment costs). For many people, this not only meant that such expenses had to come out of other income, but also contributed to bad employment practices, such as employing assistants on a cash-in-hand basis and failing to take out the appropriate insurance. Hardly surprisingly, such issues were of particular concern to organisations such as the United Kingdom Home Care Association, which expressed its fears that the subsequent introduction of direct payments might not take into account the full costs of overheads and the responsibilities incurred by becoming an employer:

> "If direct payments are going to be extended through legislation, then we have to make sure that they are not merely a back door way of reducing the cost of care." (quoted in Bond, 1996, p 20)

Since direct payments were formally implemented in April 1997, there has been ongoing concern about the hidden costs that managing payments may entail. In Scotland, many direct payment calculations do not appear to include National Insurance, sickness pay and contingency money (Witcher et al, 2000). In Staffordshire, a start up payment of £25 to cover advertising costs, stationery, postage, telephone and travel expenses was welcomed by some recipients, but criticised by others as being inadequate:

> "An initial newspaper advert was placed and £25 did not cover the costs."

> "The money allowed for advertising needs to be reassessed. You cannot advertise in the local press for less than £80. Supermarkets often refuse to put in what they consider to be job applications on their advertising boards." (Leece, 2000, p 40)

Another key concern is the level of payments which local authorities choose to make. Since this sum is discretionary, it tends to vary considerably from area to area, and the amount of support which direct payment users receive is very much a 'postcode lottery'. In Scotland, hourly payments for PAs range from £3.60 to £11.64, and some authorities have no mechanisms for paying enhanced rates for antisocial hours or for workers with additional skills (Witcher et al, 2000). Elsewhere, there is a tendency for eligibility criteria to get tighter and tighter, squeezing direct payment packages and allowing less and less time for specified activities (Hasler, 1999).

Charges can also vary, making some direct payment packages non-viable. Although a typical charge is thought to be around £15 a week, some authorities impose charges of up to 75% of the service cost if the individual's income is more than £50 above Income Support level (Age Concern, 1998; McCurry, 1999). Such is the level of concern about variations in charging practices across the country that significant changes have been announced by the government (DoH, 2001g, h) following considerable controversy and a critical report by the Audit Commission (1999). Overall, NCIL's *The rough guide to managing personal assistants* is adamant that insufficient payments are a central obstacle to successful direct payment schemes:

> Some of the difficulties described in this book could be sorted out by a more substantial Direct Payment. Without enough money independent living becomes stressful and in some circumstances almost too stressful.... Money is one of the key factors in the crusade. It is both liberator and jailer and we have to resist all attempts to minimise care packages and maximise charging. If we fail then we will be in big trouble. We will have no money to pay for the other parts of our lives (mortgages, children, vehicles) or to pay for the other mammoth costs associated with significant impairment. (Vasey, 2000, p 10)

To overcome the dangers of inadequate payments, the role of assessment is crucial and detailed guidance is available from the PSI/NCIL (Hasler et al, 1999) and from the Chartered Institute of Public Finance and Accountancy (CIPFA) (1998). For Hasler et al (1999), assessments should be holistic, needs-led, flexible and based on choice, independence and self-assessment. After this, the resultant care plan can be used as a template for costing a direct payments package, retaining sufficient flexibility to take account of inevitable fluctuations and adjustments week by week. Payments will need to include basic wages and a range of additional payments/costs (see Box 47). For CIPFA (1998), local authorities can use their knowledge of independent sector prices to help

Box 47: Costing a direct payments package

Basic wages:	These will vary in different areas of the country and specialist skills will attract higher rates of pay.
Unsocial hours:	Payments will need to take into account antisocial hours, sleep overs and public holidays.
Essential on-costs:	National Insurance, liability insurance, holiday and sick pay.
Recommended costs:	Training time, emergency cover, enhanced pay for Bank Holidays, travel and administration costs.
Contingencies:	Maternity pay or pooled funds to be drawn on as needed.

Overall, it is estimated that essential and recommended on-costs add a total of 30 to 40 per cent to the basic wages payment. (Hasler et al, 1999, pp 63-6)

them determine direct payment levels. Where users intend to employ their own staff, authorities may find it more appropriate to use their own in-house costs as a guide (including hourly salary costs and overheads). Authorities may also wish to make start-up grants to cover expenses associated with attending training courses and inductions.

A further financial difficulty concerns the monitoring processes which local authorities establish to ensure that direct payments are being spent correctly. Throughout the campaign for direct payments, there was widespread concern about the financial implications of making payments to individual disabled people (see Chapter Three), and many subsequent direct payment schemes have included clearly defined monitoring procedures to ensure that money is spent appropriately and efficiently. In many ways, this attention to financial detail is to be commended because it enables the local authority to audit its expenditure effectively, and protects disabled people against accusations of fraud or of misusing their payments. However, there is also a danger that monitoring processes can become overly bureaucratic, acting as a disincentive to take up direct payments (see Box 48). To prevent this from happening, PSI/NCIL recommend that monitoring should be proportionate to the minimum requirements to protect the liabilities both of the disabled person and of the local authority (Hasler et al, 1998). This should only include setting up a separate bank account and providing copies of time sheets and bank statements – anything more may be considered excessive.

As a result, organisations like NCIL have been critical of financial guidance issued by CIPFA (1998), which is deemed to be unnecessarily complex and obtrusive, failing to take account of the expertise of disabled people who have been running their own payment schemes for many years (see NCIL, ndd and Box 48). While most disabled people will want to demonstrate that they have

Box 48: CIPFA guidance

NCIL has great concerns over some of the guidance offered by CIPFA.... As this organisation's advice is viewed by [local authority social services departments] as sacrosanct, any departure from their approach is met with almost total resistance. Direct Payment Support Schemes have contacted NCIL to complain that CIPFA monitoring and accounting arrangements are far too bureaucratic and complex for 'users' and social service practitioners to use practically on a day to day basis. The procedures are highly intrusive and burdensome, putting many people off the idea of managing a payment scheme.... Disabled people's established Independent Living Schemes have developed accounting and audit procedures for Direct or 'Third Party' Payments over a considerable number of years. They are therefore in a position to demonstrate highly 'workable' procedures which fully meet legal and public accountability requirements. Unfortunately CIPFA failed to involve such a body of expertise when they compiled their material. (NCIL, ndd, p 5)

spent their payments correctly, this must also be balanced against the underlying feeling which some direct payment recipients have that social services staff do not trust them and that they have to account to others for everything they do (Hasler, 1999; Maglajlic et al, 2000).

A final financial barrier to overcome is the tendency of some local authorities to impose cost ceilings on direct payment packages. Highlighted by organisations such as Age Concern (1998), NCIL (ndd) and Values Into Action (Holman and Bewley, 1999), the practice of limiting care packages through cost ceilings has been criticised by the government, who feels that financial ceilings may result in premature admissions to residential care (DoH, 1998a). Cost ceilings have also been opposed by a number of disability campaigners, who have argued that limiting the amount of community-based care available to disabled people contradicts the fundamental tenets of the Independent Living Movement:

> We do not support the use of cash ceilings, as we feel that they are entirely incompatible with needs led assessment. (NCIL, ndd, p 6)

> Many local authorities operate a cost ceiling as a way of controlling their community care budget. In some this is a guideline to care managers, in others it is a straightjacket. In authorities operating a rigid cost ceiling, people whose care needs exceed a set amount are directed to residential care.... People in residential care lead 'unnecessarily isolated and restricted lives'. They are unable to take paid work and, in all but a few cases, are unable to contribute to their local communities. Within the disability movement, campaigners have been arguing that it is both inefficient and inhumane to force people into residential care because of lack of funds for community-based support. The resulting waste of human potential is a poor use of national resources, as well as personally damaging to the people concerned. (Hasler, 1997, p 13)

> People generally want to live in their own homes if they can, and admission to institutional care ... can lead to lower self-confidence and a decline in activity. Yet the evidence is that many authorities are setting a financial ceiling on their domiciliary care packages, ... which can lead to premature admissions to care homes when care at home would have been more suitable. (DoH, 1998a, p 14)

The exploitation of women?

It is an inescapable fact that most personal care in the UK and in many other countries is provided by women, who are typically poorly paid and may have substantial family commitments (Balloch et al, 1999; Abbott, 2000). In terms of family/informal care, research suggests that there are 5.7 million carers in Britain, 58% of whom are women (DoH, 2000f, p 15). While there are more male carers than was previously expected, women are more likely than men to carry the main responsibility for caring, provide more hours of care and are more likely to be assisting with personal care (Arber and Ginn, 1995a; Twigg, 1998; DoH, 2000f). This is particularly the case in intergenerational caring, which is once again associated more with women than with men (Twigg, 1998).

There is now an extensive body of literature to suggest that caring may have major (and often negative) physical, financial, social and psychological consequences, not just in the short term, but also in the long run after the caring relationship has finished (see, for example, Goodman, 1986; McLaughlin and Ritchie, 1994; Arber and Ginn, 1995b; Drew, 1995; Hancock and Jarvis, 1995; Carmichael and Charles, 1998; Henwood, 1998; Hoffman and Mitchell, 1998). Against this background, the restriction on using direct payments to employ close relatives means that female family members providing care for disabled family members will continue to do so free of charge, without being able to receive a wage for their work via their family member's direct payments (see Chapter Three). This is a complex issue, but it is possible that the government's decision to prevent the employment of close relatives may have been motivated by the assumption that female family members should already be providing care free of charge and that paying them for their work would make direct payments far too expensive. By preventing family members from being employed by direct payment recipients, therefore, the government may be contributing to the exploitation of women.

In terms of paid carers, gender issues are once again significant. During the 1970s, data collected by the Department of Health and Social Security suggested that women formed 64% of social workers, 70% of residential home care assistants and 83% of social work assistants, with most management positions falling to men (Howe, 1986, pp 23-4). By 1987, social services departments were identified as the most occupationally segregated area of the welfare state, with women comprising 87.2% of the social services workforce (Hallett, 1989, p 33). In addition to practising as social workers and social work assistants, women were thought to make up around three quarters of the 'manual workforce', receiving low rates of pay and working as home helps, domestic staff and wardens of sheltered housing (Jones, 1989). By 1990, 86.5% of the social services workforce were women, with the majority employed as part-time workers (Davis, 1996, p 122). Once again, social services departments were found to be "pyramid organisations in which women dominate the base and men outnumber women at the peak" – a feature of social work which had not changed significantly since the creation of local authority social services departments in 1971 (Davis, 1996, p 123). During the 1990s, research carried out by the National Institute for Social Work suggested that women represented well over 80% of the social services workforce in England, Scotland and Northern Ireland, often combining their work with substantial family commitments (Balloch et al, 1999). Perhaps unsurprisingly, stress levels were higher for women with young children who worked full time than for their male colleagues (Ginn and Sandell, 1997), and women were more likely to be employed at lower grades and at lower management levels than men. By 2001, a Unison survey of 3,047 home carers found that more than 97% were women, receiving low pay, often working unsocial hours, suffering from back pain and finding their work increasingly stressful (Unison, 2001). 'Care work', in short, is a gendered activity.

Against this background, it is possible that the majority of PAs employed by direct payment recipients will be women (although this must remain conjecture until further research is undertaken into the background and type of people who become PAs). We have already seen how some direct payment schemes can create financial difficulties for disabled people due to their failure to take into account hidden costs and due to the emphasis on the cost-effective use of public resources. Viewed from this angle, could direct payments result in the greater exploitation of women? Certainly, this is the stance adopted by commentators such as Ungerson (1997), who argues that direct payments may generate hardship for poorly paid women and other vulnerable groups. Rather than an *internal market* or *quasi-market*, Ungerson likens direct payments to a "flea market" in which everyone involved is on low incomes, the services delivered are not highly valued, some activity is illegal and where it is possible, in some situations, to find a particular 'bargain' or 'treasure' who will work well beyond market and contractual requirements. Underlying this is a clear gender issue which Ungerson is quick to highlight:

> Although we know next to nothing about the kinds of people that work as personal assistants – except anecdotally – one can begin to guess who will come forward. Many of them will be women wishing to fit casual work, at unsociable hours, around the calls of their domestic lives and generate an income for themselves and their children. Some will be students in need of money to support their education, but will be able to work in flexible packets of time. Others will be seeking housing solutions to their accommodation problems; some will be on benefit looking to enhance their incomes, either legally up to the earnings disregard for their particular benefit, or illegally beyond their benefit rules. Although direct payments will be 'monitored' by

> local authorities to ensure they are being spent properly in care services, there is nothing to suggest ... that the market itself will be carefully policed. Hence, informal and illegal contractual arrangements, where the workers have no employment rights of any kind, are likely to develop. (1997, p 50)

Although Ungerson was writing before direct payments were formally implemented in April 1997, research findings do suggest that her concerns may have some weight. In 1993, a study of the experiences of disabled service users found that some payment recipients made 'cash-in-hand' payments to PAs due to the inadequacy of the money they received (Morris, 1993a). Around the same time, Zarb and Nadash (1994) found that around 60% of respondents felt that the wages which they paid to PAs were too low. Many did not pay their workers holiday pay[1] and a few people made payments 'cash-in-hand'. Should they receive any increase in funding, many people signalled their intention to increase their workers' wages and/or increase the number of hours worked (see Table 11). This led the researchers to the conclusion that "although some people employing their own workers feel they have had to cut corners in the way they organise their support, this is invariably out of necessity rather than by choice" (Zarb and Nadash, 1994, p 42), a sentiment echoed by the BCODP (John Evans, quoted in George, 1994a, p 15). Other studies have suggested that the rates of pay which direct payment recipients are able to offer do not reflect the types of work that PAs are expected to undertake nor the skills that they may require (Glendinning et al, 2000a, b, c). Similar concerns have also been raised elsewhere in Europe, as a French director of social services has acknowledged:

> "Disabled people are happier and more independent [receiving direct payments], but the position of employees is fragile, with less training, less security and irregular hours of work." (quoted in Wellard, 1999, p 23)

In response to issues such as these, disabled researchers such as Morris (1997) have emphasised that the majority of disabled employers do not give 'cash-in-hand'. Even those that do are probably no different from many non-disabled people who purchase services such as cleaning and childminding on an informal

Table 11: How people would spend an increase in payments

	Number	%
Increase weekly hours	14	37
Increase workers' pay	13	34
Increase workers' hours and pay	6	16
Pay workers' tax/National Insurance	5	13
Total	**38**	**100**

Source: Zarb and Nadash (1994, p 42)

basis, while the concept of making direct payments to qualifying individuals is similar to the child benefit system:

> How many people pay someone to do their housework, and how many pay cash in hand? Those of us who do so may think of ourselves as good employers: we may pay at or above the local 'going rate', some of us may pay sick pay, bank holidays and holidays (I suspect more will not), but most of us don't deduct tax and national insurance or pay the employers' national insurance contribution. In fact, most of us would find it hard to get a cleaner if we insisted on anything other than a 'cash in hand' relationship. Does this mean that we are exploiting these low-paid women?... The child benefit system is ... a system of cash payments made to individuals. I wonder how many mothers spend their child benefit in parts of the informal economy or on goods and services in the formal economy made or delivered by low-paid workers. Yet presumably Clare Ungerson would not wish to use this to question the value of the child benefit system. (Morris, 1997, pp 58-60)

For Morris, direct payments represent an opportunity to break down the stereotypes which disabled people have traditionally faced and establish their status as citizens, able to use cash payments in order to do what they want rather than what professional workers think they want. As a result, Morris feels that social researchers have a moral responsibility to collaborate with what she sees as a civil rights movement concerned with people's right to choice and control over their own lives. While both arguments (Morris and Ungerson) are persuasive, a way forward would surely seem to lie in the findings of Zarb and Nadash (1994) that many disabled people would want to pay higher wages if they received higher payments. Ultimately, the risk of exploiting women may lie not so much in the concept of direct payments itself, as in the way that many schemes are operationalised by social services departments, the restriction on employing family members and the inadequate levels of payments that are sometimes made (as previously discussed).

Risk

As pressure for direct payments mounted in the early 1990s, a key feature of the government's initial refusal to implement such a scheme was the argument that making cash payments to disabled service users would leave them at risk. This was rejected by disabled campaigners (who argued that they were already at risk from substandard local authority services), and ultimately defeated. However, even after the successful implementation of direct payments in many parts of the country, concerns about risk continue to surface (Burrows, 2001; George, 2001) and do raise doubts about direct payments as currently conceptualised.

In most of the literature on direct payments, the issue of risk is either downplayed or rejected outright. In a Department of Health (1998c) promotional video, one commentator is adamant that the risk associated with direct payments is minimal and that taking risks is a central feature of being in control of one's own services. A similar argument is also put forward by NCIL, who emphasise that taking risks is an important citizen right and that the empowerment offered by direct payments can actually reduce risks by making people more in control of their lives, and enabling them to avoid abusive situations (see Box 49).

Box 49: Risk versus empowerment

Protection from abuse is linked to empowerment in that it is the common experience of disabled people that the more we are in control of our lives, and the support we need to lead them, the less likely we are to find ourselves in abusive situations.
It must be recognised that historically, disabled people's freedom of movement, choice and control has been regularly denied or curtailed in the name of 'safety'.... Disabled people must be given the same rights to take risks as all citizens. (NCIL, 1999, pp 4, 8)

Although these are persuasive arguments, the issue of risk is one that does need to be addressed if direct payment schemes are to be successful. While organisations such as NCIL are correct to suggest that risk has traditionally been used to restrict disabled people's liberties, this does not mean that risk can be ignored or that action to increase safety should be overlooked. As a practical illustration of the risks which employing a PA can entail, Vasey's (2000) *The rough guide to managing personal assistants* describes a number of situations in which PA users have found themselves employing exploitative or dishonest workers (see also Box 50 for a more extreme example).

Box 50: Dialling 999

In the October 2000 edition of the BCODP Personal Assistants Users' Newsletter, one woman described how her PA arrived for an evening shift drunk. The PA had been in the woman's employment for eleven months without having a day off or being late once, and said that her drunkenness was due to domestic pressures. Although the woman wanted to give her PA the benefit of the doubt, it soon became apparent that the PA was so drunk that it would be dangerous for her to assist the woman. When the woman tried to send her away, however, the PA became abusive and refused to leave the woman's house. When the woman tried to phone a friend, the PA tried to wrestle the telephone off her. After the woman's friend had called the police the PA eventually left. Since the woman had placed a clause in her contract that PAs can be instantly dismissed if they arrive for work under the influence of alcohol or drugs, she was able to terminate the PA's employment immediately. (Bailey, 2000)

As part of its modernisation programme for public services, the New Labour government issued a White Paper emphasising the need to protect "vulnerable people" from abuse and to change the way that social services are provided and regulated:

> The present regulatory arrangements are incomplete and patchy, and the Government will replace them with a system that is modern, independent and dependable. Taken together with the establishment of the General Social Care Council [to regulate the training and conduct of social care workers], these reforms will put in place new systems for ensuring that when people receive care it is safe and of high quality ... and that the staff on whom they rely have the training, skills and standards that are necessary for the work they do. (DoH, 1998a, p 64)

In pursuit of these aims, the government has introduced regional Commissions for Care Standards to regulate and inspect residential and domiciliary care providers. At the same time, the new General Social Care Council will register certain types of social care worker and set standards of conduct. While commentators such as NCIL have welcomed many of these policies, they have emphasised that disabled people should be allowed to take risks on a par with non-disabled people and that greater regulation should not restrict the rights of disabled people to employ PAs of their choice, regardless of training or registration (NCIL, 1999). Thus, direct payments seem to raise something of a dilemma in which safeguarding disabled people against abuse has to be balanced against the right of individuals to exercise choice and control over their own lives. Although this may prove a difficult balance to achieve, there are two key issues to highlight:

- One possible solution may be for local authorities and central government to ensure that there is adequate funding available for support mechanisms so that PA users can consider issues of risk in advance and develop preventative strategies. With the correct support, disabled people beginning to receive direct payments could adopt employment practices that minimise risk (such as not giving out personal contact details in advertisements, asking appropriate questions at interviews, following up references and so on). When problems arise, direct payment recipients could share their experiences and develop their own solutions through peer support.
- Provided that sensible precautions are taken, it is difficult to see how receiving direct payments could be any more risky than receiving direct services. In Box 50, for example, the disabled person would have been just as vulnerable to physical assault had a local authority employee arrived drunk as she was with a PA that she employed herself. In this particular case, the PA had worked for the woman for eleven months, had shown herself to be reliable and was presumably a trusted worker. As a result, the fact that the PA was employed through a direct payment rather than by the local authority or a private agency seems to be irrelevant, and this incident could presumably have occurred just as easily if the woman was receiving directly provided services.

'Offloading troublemakers'

Although there is currently no direct evidence, there is a danger that 'difficult' service users may be encouraged to receive direct payments so that local authority services do not have to have ongoing contact with them. In this scenario, 'difficult' is often a shorthand term to refer to potentially violent or verbally/ sexually abusive users, and the suggestion is that some authorities may be tempted to 'offload' such 'troublemakers'. Of course, it was precisely for this reason that disabled people welcomed the emphasis of the 1996 Community Care (Direct Payments) Act and subsequent guidance on disabled people being 'willing' to receive payments – a requirement that should stop local authorities from making payments to alleged 'troublemakers' without their consent. However, the example cited in Box 51 does suggest that at least one local authority may be relatively proactive in recommending direct payments for service users it feels are a threat to its own staff. Although this whole issue must remain conjecture without further research, it does raise questions about the possible use and abuse of direct payments.

Box 51: 'Offloading troublemakers'

In one local authority, the social services department has found it difficult to reconcile the rights of service users with the health and safety of its staff. Where users are deemed to be violent and aggressive, the department is very aware that it has a duty to meet the needs of users while at the same time protecting its employees. In such a situation, legal advice suggests that the department could try to discharge its responsibilities by purchasing care from a private agency. If private care is not available for any particular reason, legal advisors have recommended that the social services department considers direct payments as a means of ensuring that an appropriate service is provided to the individual service user without jeopardising the safety of workers or exposing them to unacceptable verbal abuse. This seems to be an abuse of the concept of direct payments, which should be based on the empowerment of disabled people and the enhancement of user choice and control, not on attempts by social services departments to 'offload troublemakers'.

Practical challenges and support mechanisms

Managing direct payments is not easy and recipients face a number of practical challenges to overcome:

- employment legislation;
- tax and National Insurance;
- accounting;
- recruitment;
- miscellaneous issues such as arranging cover and the training/support needs of PAs.

Although many of these issues are dealt with in much greater detail in Chapter Nine, it is important that service users and their social workers are aware of the practical challenges that direct payments can raise and are clear about the way in which these challenges are to be overcome. Unless these issues are carefully considered, the result can be a situation in which service users unused to managing their own payments may be left to struggle on alone without adequate support. At best, this will be stressful for the individuals concerned and may prejudice them against direct payments in the future. At worst, it could lead to a breakdown in care arrangements, with potential financial and legal implications for the service user and/or their social services department.

Throughout the current literature on direct payments, the need for adequate support structures is an almost constant theme (see, for example, Simpson with Campbell, 1996; Dunnicliff, 1999; Hasler et al, 1999; Glendinning et al, 2000c), and the absence of such support can be a major barrier that is difficult to overcome (Witcher et al, 2000). This is recognised by Department of Health guidance (1997a, 2000a) and has also been highlighted through evaluations undertaken by the Social Services Inspectorate (Fruin, 2000, p 16). In six authorities where direct payments were in place, users were found to need assistance in starting to receive payments and managing them on an ongoing basis, both in terms of administrative issues and psychological support. This was sometimes provided by a local disability organisation, by other voluntary agencies or by specialist social services staff, although there was no evidence of peer support or self-help groups in any of the authorities concerned. In other areas of the country, some authorities have also sought to make detailed support arrangement before direct payments are introduced. Thus, the support offered by a voluntary organisation in Staffordshire was welcomed by direct payment recipients (Leece, 2000), while Norfolk social services established a very structured support system which offered users a range of choices depending on their needs and wishes (Dawson, 2000, pp 10-11):

- Option 1: Self-management (with training and peer support available from a local disability organisation).
- Option 2: Assisted management (where an agent assists the user to manage their payments, with training and peer support once again available).
- Option 3: Assisted management – Independent Living Project (where a social services project provides payroll services, with training and peer support once again available).

Nowhere is the importance of adequate support more apparent than in the PSI/NCIL guidance for local authorities seeking to implement and manage direct payment schemes (Hasler et al, 1999). To emphasise the centrality of effective support mechanisms, the guidance notes that in areas where disabled people are successfully managing direct payments, there is always an established support service to assist them:

> Support services are perhaps the most fundamental part of a successful direct payments scheme. The purpose of direct payments support services is to ensure that adequate advice, information and support are available to disabled people so that they may feel confident to undertake the complexities of using direct payments to employ and manage their own staff. Such support also ensures that individuals using a direct payment are operating legally and efficiently. The support service has to be properly funded and responsive. (Hasler et al, 1999, p 11)

Although they may have different names (self-operated care schemes, personal assistance support schemes, centres for independent living, independent/integrated living schemes), all support services should include four core features:

- peer support (so that disabled people can share information and experiences, develop practical solutions to problems and support each other);
- information (covering all aspects of independent living and direct payments, available in a range of formats and languages);
- advice and/or advocacy (to assist disabled people to manage their payments and find solutions to any problems);
- training (about independent living, recruiting staff, time management, building relationships with staff, legal responsibilities and administrative duties) (Hasler et al, 1999, pp 12-15).

In addition to this, some support schemes may offer a payroll service, employ staff on behalf of the service user and hold registers of PAs. To be truly effective, support mechanisms require adequate funding (to cover both start-up costs and ongoing work). For further information, regularly updated lists of Personal Assistance Support Schemes are available from NCIL (2000b).

Despite the undoubted need for adequate support mechanisms, there is evidence to suggest that some direct payment recipients may not always receive the assistance they require to make their care packages work successfully. In two audits by the Social Services Inspectorate, for example, the local authorities concerned had attempted to identify disability organisations to take on a support role, but were unable to find any agencies available/willing to do so (Fruin, 2000, pp 16-17). Elsewhere, some support schemes have found it difficult to survive due to funding difficulties (Hasler et al, 1999, p 23), and some direct payments schemes are felt to be floundering because the local authority is using social workers to advise service users, rather than organisations of disabled people (McCurry, 1999). While some support is presumably better than none at all, there are concerns that many social workers are not trained in issues such as employment legislation or financial management and feel stressed about having to offer this support in addition to their normal case loads. Certainly, this is an issue that has been highlighted time and time again by organisations of disabled people, and one which has been re-emphasised following the various extensions of direct payments to new user groups (NCIL, 1999, p 4):

> NCIL welcomes the extension of Direct Payments ... but are very concerned that a budget has not been forthcoming to develop an infrastructure of support to new payment users. Currently, such support schemes are funded from existing Social Services budgets, which we are told are insufficient to meet the need of essential services, let alone new development.

If direct payments really are to be successful, they need to be based on well-established support mechanisms which are valued and adequately funded by local authorities:

> It is very important to see independent living support services as part of community care and not just an optional extra. Because support services are a vital component of implementing direct payments, local authorities need to recognise their importance, and give them a high priority when determining budget allocation. (Hasler et al, 1999, p 24)

SUMMARY

Despite the positive aspects of direct payments emphasised in Chapter Seven, payments (as currently conceived) may also bring a number of disadvantages which need to be acknowledged and overcome. Introduced by a Conservative government committed to rolling back the frontiers of the welfare state, there is a potential contradiction between the emphasis of the Independent Living Movement on choice and control, and a government agenda influenced by flawed notions of consumerism. Implemented against the backdrop of attempts to curtail public expenditure, direct payment schemes may not have received sufficient funding, resulting in financial difficulties for some local authorities, inadequate payments and support arrangements, low wages for PAs and the potential exploitation of women. Other difficulties include the possibility of a shift in the health and social care divide, the need to balance empowerment against risk, and the danger of local authorities viewing direct payments as a means of 'offloading troublemakers'.

Throughout, a key barrier has been the attitude and practices of frontline social workers, who occupy an important gatekeeping role and can sometimes hinder rather than facilitate the dissemination of information about direct payments. All this is not to suggest that direct payments are a 'bad thing' – on the contrary the authors believe that the advantages of direct payments far outweigh the potential disadvantages. However, it is important that some of the negative features of direct payments are identified and challenged so that disabled people are adequately informed about the options open to them before they make decisions about their care arrangements and so that the system can be improved.

Note

[1] At the time of Zarb and Nadash's study (1994) holiday pay was optional rather than mandatory.

NINE

Practical issues

Chapter Eight concluded by outlining some of the key practical challenges facing disabled people who are contemplating receiving direct payments and the importance of careful planning to ensure that these challenges can be satisfactorily overcome. Significant issues include:

- employment legislation;
- tax and National Insurance;
- accounting;
- recruitment;
- a range of miscellaneous issues.

While this chapter focuses in more detail on some of the practicalities of managing a direct payment, it is important to avoid the trap of assuming that disabled people are unable to rise to these challenges and overcome the obstacles in the way of independent living. As we have already seen, the very implementation of direct payments was in large part the result of longstanding pressure from groups of disabled people committed to removing the barriers to independent living enshrined in the 1948 National Assistance Act. After the 1996 Community Care (Direct Payments) Act came into force in 1997, more and more schemes have developed, often supported by Centres for Independent Living, and disabled people have proved extremely capable of rising to the practical issues that direct payments raise. Although managing direct payments may be difficult at times, this should not stop disabled people from attempting to do so. Above all, this is the resounding message that emerges from NCIL's *The rough guide to managing personal assistants*:

> Direct Payments really represent a golden opportunity for disabled people. They are the means by which we close the chapter of disability history called 'Institutions' and move on to the part of the story where we get a crack at living just like everybody else. With the right facilitation any disabled person, whatever their impairment, can take control and be free to get on with life. It all seems so simple, but of course like so many things it is just a bit more complicated than it first appears.... We are all wrestling with the same issues. Everybody finds it an effort, at least some of the time, because it is basically management work that we are involved in here and management is rarely easy. In business, managers are paid large sums and then often do it badly. We get paid nothing and cannot afford to fail, not only because our living arrangements will instantly be in tatters, but because there is a view widely held by the powers that be that we are not up to the job. This book [*The*

rough guide] is a celebration of disabled people's undoubted ability to get on with a difficult job in order to get a life. (Vasey, 2000, pp 7-8)

Employment legislation

Although disabled people can choose to use their direct payments in a number of ways, many opt to employ their own workers since this gives them maximum control over their care arrangements (Lakey, 1994; Glendinning et al, 1999c). However, by becoming an employer, the direct payment recipient is taking on a number of legal responsibilities and has to be aware of a number of rules and regulations concerning their duties to their staff. While employment law and practices continue to evolve, key issues to consider include (Simpson with Campbell, 1996; ILSA, 1998; Hampshire Centre for Independent Living, 2000):

- anti-discriminatory legislation such as the 1975 Sex Discrimination Act and the 1976 Race Relations Act, as well as European Union regulations such as the Directive on Equal Treatment in Employment and Occupation (European Union, 2000);
- the provisions of the 1996 Employment Act;
- redundancy and unfair dismissal;
- rights to maternity leave and maternity pay;
- rights to sick pay;
- regulations concerning the number of hours that PAs may work;
- the minimum wage;
- health and safety issues;
- employers' Liability Insurance and Public Liability Insurance to protect against injury to PAs or to others.

Whenever employment issues are mentioned with regard to direct payments, many local authorities immediately think of what has become known as the 'South Lanarkshire' case (see Box 52).

In fact, the South Lanarkshire case has much less relevance for direct payments than may at first be apparent. Following the initial reporting of the tribunal, a series of more detailed commentaries by Values Into Action (Bewley, 2000a, b, c) has suggested that the "tribunal ruling has no legal relevance for direct payments" (Bewley, 2000b, p 3). Above all, Bewley emphasises that neither Ian Brown nor the disabled person who lived with him, were receiving direct payments. Instead, their care package was 95% funded through an independent living service and 5% by the ILF. While there was some confusion as to the exact nature of the service, it is clear that it was not part of a direct payments package (Bewley, 2000c):

- The independent living service appears to have been an arms-length organisation, funded and run by the social services department.
- The service was introduced before direct payments were legalised in 1996.

Box 52: The South Lanarkshire case

In 1999, an employment tribunal case concerning an allegation of sexual harassment was reported in the social work press (*Community Care*, 1999; Hunter, 1999; McCurry, 1999). While at first glance the case appeared to concern a female PA who took out a case against her disabled employer, the tribunal ruled that South Lanarkshire Council, not the disabled person, was the employer and therefore liable. Although the reporting of the case did not make it clear what sort of funding the disabled person in question was receiving, much of the commentary surrounding the case seemed to imply that local authorities may be responsible for the employees of all direct payment recipients. Hardly surprisingly, this prompted significant concerns around the country from social services departments anxious about the legal and financial implications of the ruling (Hunter, 1999).

> **Case threatens direct payments**
>
> The recent employment tribunal ruling concerning a personal assistant and her disabled employer is open to a variety of interpretations, and has raised the temperature of the debate over direct payments. The controversy centres around the case of Lorna Smith, a care worker from South Lanarkshire in Scotland, who worked for two years as a personal assistant to Ian Brown, a man with multiple disabilities. Smith claimed she had been sexually harassed by Brown. However, in a landmark judgement, the tribunal ruled that South Lanarkshire Council rather than Brown should be regarded as Smith's employer and thereby liable for damages.... Social services chiefs are deeply concerned by the idea that local authorities are to be held responsible for the industrial relations of disabled employers who have opted out of local authority care. (Hunter, 1999, p 10)

- Disabled people did not directly control the money.
- The social services department was heavily involved in writing and placing the job advertisement, producing employment papers, interviewing and training the PA.
- A third party (a disability organisation) organised the rota for the PAs, received weekly timesheets, agreed annual leave and dealt with any complaints by the PAs.

As a result of these factors, the tribunal chairman ruled that South Lanarkshire Council was the PA's employer, and this decision was upheld on appeal. With hindsight, it seems clear that the scheme in operation in South Lanarkshire was not a direct payments scheme at all, and that the case should not be used by social services departments as an excuse for restricting access to direct payments. On the contrary, all the available evidence suggests that the complexities of the South Lanarkshire case could have been avoided if there had been more clarity, and should encourage local authorities to extend direct payments to a greater number of people as a means of putting their independent living schemes on a clearer, unambiguous footing.

In seeking to keep abreast of their responsibilities as employers, direct payment recipients can make use of a range of sources of information. At a local level, many support schemes will be able to provide up-to-date advice on employment legislation and may also be able to offer practical assistance with particular aspects of employing a PA (such as help with writing contracts and pay-roll schemes). At a national level, specialist information may be available from agencies such as the Inland Revenue, the Health and Safety Executive (HSE) and the Advisory, Conciliation and Arbitration Service (ACAS) (see the Appendix for contact details). Useful sources of written information include:

- The New Employer's Starter Pack from the Inland Revenue (nd) contains information about tax, National Insurance, sick pay, maternity pay and other relevant literature. Further information is available from the Inland Revenue Helpline (advertised in the Starter Pack), which has a Typetalk service for disabled people.
- ACAS publishes a series of advisory leaflets on employment-related issues.
- The Equal Opportunities Commission and the Commission for Racial Equality publish information on a range of topics concerning anti-discriminatory employment practice.
- The HSE produces a number of information leaflets on issues such as health and safety at work and manual handling (see, for example, HSE, 1995, 2000).
- Disability organisations publish a range of useful guides which contain information about employment issues (see, for example, NCIL, 1988; Dunne with Hoyle, 1992; ILSA, 1998). A sample contract and information regarding how to dismiss a PA are also available on the NCIL website (see Appendix).

Tax and National Insurance

By employing PAs, direct payment recipients may become legally responsible for deducting tax under the Pay as You Earn (PAYE) scheme and National Insurance contributions from their workers' pay. Depending on the income of PAs, the disabled employer may also be liable for Employer's National Insurance contributions. This can be a difficult issue for new direct payment recipients, and one that has generated considerable concern and publicity in the past following a number of high profile cases. Thus, while the Community Care (Direct Payments) Bill was being debated, some commentators were already citing the example of two disabled people receiving ILF payments who accumulated debts of £6,000 and £8,000 respectively by making payments to the Inland Revenue at the wrong level or misunderstanding their responsibilities (Bond, 1996). After the implementation of the 1996 Community Care (Direct Payments) Act, one social services department was able to negotiate with the local tax office for all PAs to work on a self-employed basis, thus reducing the responsibilities placed on the disabled person. However, this solution seemed to cause concern during an inspection by the Social Services Inspectorate, who were worried about what would happen if the tax office changed its view, and about difficulties that could arise in relation to the status of the employee if a dispute went to the employment tribunal (DoH/SSI, 1999d).

Despite the anxiety which tax and National Insurance can cause, making the correct deductions can become a routine task with correct information and appropriate support. In some areas of the country, direct payment support schemes may even run a payroll service that handles tax and National Insurance issues on behalf of disabled people (see, for example, ILSA, 1998), although there is usually a charge for this service and the cost should be considered when designing a direct payments package and calculating the level of payments to be made (Simpson with Campbell, 1996). To ensure that direct payment recipients are adequately supported, the Disablement Income Group recommends that all advice should include the following (Simpson with Campbell, 1996, p 9):

- A clear explanation of the difference between employing people on a PAYE system or using self-employed PAs.
- If PAs are to work on a self-employed basis, users should be advised to ensure they have written confirmation from the local tax office of the employment status of the PA.
- Support and training on running a PAYE system.
- If an employee earns less than the National Insurance threshold, users should be advised to ask the employee to sign a form to declare that they are not employed by someone else.
- The support worker should ask the local tax office to inform them of all relevant information, if necessary by means of a visit.

In addition to advice from direct payment support schemes and the local tax office, information is available from sources such as the Inland Revenue (nd) New Employer's Starter Pack (referred to above).

Accounting

As noted in Chapter Eight, receiving direct payments brings with it additional responsibilities in terms of accounting for the way in which the payment is spent and keeping financial records. Like tax and National Insurance, this can be a daunting task, but one that can be simplified and made more manageable with the correct information and support (BCODP, 1995). While different direct payment schemes will have different financial requirements, key themes are likely to include (see Box 53 for practical examples):

- the need for a separate bank account so that direct payment recipients can distinguish their payments from their personal money;
- the need to keep regular records regarding income and expenditure;
- the need to submit regular financial statements to the social services department.

Box 53: Hampshire direct payments

In Hampshire, direct payment recipients are required to:

- Open a separate bank account for their direct payments, providing social services with the sort code and account number.
- Complete and submit quarterly financial statements, including income, expenditure and balance carried forward.
- Keep records of income and expenditure. (Hampshire Centre for Independent Living, 2000)

In the west of England, ILSA (1998) publishes examples of relevant financial and administrative forms including:

Time sheets
Employee personnel sheet
Holiday form
Record of attendance
Bank reconciliation sheets
Quarterly financial statement
Weekly rota
Sickness absence form
Money paid into/out of bank account

Although official financial guidance has been criticised by organisations of disabled people (see Chapter Eight), other sources of information and assistance are available. For example:

- Hampshire Centre for Independent Living (2000) provides an advice sheet on record keeping with sample forms.
- Support schemes such as that run by the West of England Centre for Integrated Living offer assistance with budgeting, financial monitoring and record keeping, providing suggested rates of pay and sample forms (ILSA, 1998).
- Guidance published by the PSI/NCIL offers advice to local authorities on making and monitoring payments (Hasler et al, 1999, pp 75-82).

Recruitment

For many direct payment recipients, recruiting staff can be a major source of difficulty and consternation. This is particularly the case in some rural areas (where population is sparse and the pool of potential workers small) and in areas of the country such as the South East where wages are relatively high and direct payment recipients are not always able to pay competitive wages. While many disabled people are able to recruit PAs by word of mouth (Morris, 1993a, pp 128-30) and through informal social networks (Dawson, 1995, 2000), this can be an area of potential concern for some disabled people otherwise interested in using direct payments to employ their own care staff.

Prior to the 1996 Community Care (Direct Payments) Act, research into the

ILF and into indirect payment schemes identified the difficulties that some disabled people found in recruiting staff. In the early 1990s, a series of interviews with ILF recipients found that around one quarter of participants reported difficulties recruiting carers (Kestenbaum, 1993b). In London, one 66-year-old woman with rheumatoid arthritis spent months trying to recruit someone to help with domestic care, advertising in shops and church magazines:

> "It was an absolute nightmare. Everybody [was] very understanding but nothing [was] forthcoming. I couldn't understand it. I couldn't believe there wasn't someone within the area that would fit in, whether morning, afternoon or evening." (Kestenbaum, 1993b, p 12)

There were also difficulties reported by people with specific needs:

- One woman and her baby (both with brittle bone disease) "frightened off" many potential carers due to the nature of their condition.
- One person with dementia was looking for a Punjabi-speaking worker.
- One man with advanced MS lived in an isolated, rural area and used an agency. Only two members of the agency's staff were able to cope with his needs (Kestenbaum, 1993b, p 13).

While trying to recruit workers, some of the disabled people questioned felt that they had been unsupported by their social workers and many were reluctant to advertise too widely for fear of publicising their vulnerability and attracting "the wrong sort of person" (Kestenbaum, 1993b, p 17). Difficulties recruiting staff were also reported by research conducted by the PSI, with 43% of payment recipients identifying problems in finding suitable workers:

> "I think any employer finds it difficult choosing the right person to come and do the job."
>
> "I am having difficulty recruiting staff at the moment. But I guess that's something I am always going to have difficulties with – recruiting staff. I wish there was somewhere you could phone up and say, have you got anyone on your books at the moment who is looking for a position? If there is, I don't know of it."
>
> "The most difficult thing is recruiting staff. I would just love to see a system where you could phone up somewhere and say, have you got something that might be suitable." (Zarb and Nadash, 1994, pp 45, 108)

After the legalisation of direct payments in 1996/97, recruitment difficulties have often persisted. In Staffordshire, two out of five direct payment recipients who responded to an evaluation of a pilot project wished to employ PAs but were unable to recruit suitable workers (Leece, 2000). In Scotland, nine out of the 12 authorities where direct payment recipients employ their own staff, or use agencies, reported that service users experienced difficulties identifying an appropriate individual or agency to meet their care needs. Key issues included low levels of pay, recruiting people of a particular age/gender, recruiting people to work a small number of hours or split shifts and finding PAs with the right characteristics for individual recipients (Witcher et al, 2000, para 2.44).

In Norfolk, direct payment recipients sometimes encountered difficulties with people not turning up to interviews and found it hard to attract people who were sufficiently flexible (Dawson, 2000). Some disabled people also found that they had a high turnover of workers (for example, where the worker was a student and left university), having to go through the difficult process of recruiting workers again and again.

Elsewhere, disabled employers may find that they have too few care hours to recruit workers on a full-time basis, that there is an insufficient supply of suitably qualified workers and that it is difficult to attract quality applicants due to low pay (Leece, 2000; Valois, 2000b). Where responses to advertisements are low, disabled people may feel that it is unrealistic to ask for minimum qualifications or experience and find themselves lowering their initial expectations about the quality of worker they are able to employ (Glendinning et al, 2000a).

Once a group of potential employees have been identified, disabled people need to ensure that they select the most appropriate person for the job. For some disabled people, this can often depend on the personality of the individuals involved rather than on previous skills or experience. Since PAs will be coming into people's homes and may be providing a range of intimate personal care tasks, it is important that the disabled employer chooses staff that he or she will be able to trust and get on with. Certainly, this was a key finding of an evaluation of the experience of ILF recipients:

> "The chemistry has to be right."
>
> "It can be very difficult [selecting the right person]. You have to think – are they physically capable of doing the care? Are you going to get on with them? Are they going to fit in with your family? – they'll be in your house seven days a week. You have to have some sort of rapport going. It doesn't work otherwise."
>
> "It comes quite hard to both of us to have someone else intruding in your own very private life and home. That's why it's very important to get the right person." (Kestenbaum, 1993b, p 12)

More recently, the importance of reliable, trustworthy PAs capable of fitting into the disabled person's lifestyle has been re-emphasised in a number of research studies and first hand accounts by disabled people (see, for example, Lakey, 1994; Zarb and Nadash, 1994; Glendinning et al, 1999c; Vasey, 2000). Despite the importance of recruiting suitable workers, finding such individuals can be difficult and disabled employers often find that they do not always make the right choice when interviewing potential staff, or that the 'right' person simply does not come forward. In one study, one disabled person felt that "for 99 frogs there was one prince" (quoted in Glendinning et al, 2000c, p 206) and cited low pay, and the relatively few hours of work that disabled people could offer PAs as key factors. Nowhere is the difficulty of recruiting staff more clearly illustrated than in NCIL's *The rough guide to managing personal assistants* (Vasey, 2000), which provides numerous examples of what can go wrong when recruiting, interviewing and selecting PAs (see Box 54).

In light of these recruitment difficulties, some disabled people have expressed a desire to employ household members and relatives as PAs (see, for example, Elkington, 1996; Age Concern, 1998; Leece, 2000). As noted in Chapter Four, this is prohibited by official guidance (DoH, 1997a, 2000a), although non-resident relatives and other people living in the same household can sometimes be employed as PAs in situations where this is the only appropriate way of securing relevant services. Whether or not direct payments should be used to employ family members is a complex issue. On the one hand, there may be a risk of family members exploiting their disabled relatives or of informal carers being pressured to give up work if direct payments could be used to employ

Box 54: Recruiting PAs

"I will never forget my feeling of total amazement when an applicant turned up on my doorstep with her Italian husband and her mother. The reason given for this was that they wanted to check me out to make sure I was genuine.... Needless to say, she did not get the job."

"Peter arrived one Saturday afternoon for an interview. A pleasant young man, immaculately dressed.... After two hours and cups of tea we were still talking.... He was asked to start the following Saturday and has never been seen from that day to this."

"I used to employ PAs directly myself, but... the standard of applicants was poor. Most who applied were women who could not get shop or factory work – generally because of unreliability."

"Being a PA user is not something I'm comfortable with or very good at. I struggle with the business of recruiting.... I am getting better as I have learnt from some bad experiences."

One PA user recalls some of the responses given to him in interviews:

> "I've healed all my clients, usually in the first week."
>
> "So I don't have to nag you then about taking your tablets and eating your food?"

(Vasey, 2000, pp 19-21, 26-7)

household members/close relatives (DoH/Scottish Office/Welsh Office/ Northern Ireland Office, 1996). At the same time, many European payment schemes permit the employment of close relatives (Halloran, 1998; Schunk, 1998; Pijl, 2000), as does the ILF (as long as the relative does not live in the same household) (ILF, 2000). Preventing the employment of family members also limits the choice which direct payments are supposed to promote (Age Concern, 1998). This is particularly problematic for people with progressive or fluctuating conditions who can experience a sudden deterioration and may want their family to care for them during one-off crisis periods or at short notice (NCIL, ndb). While there are no easy answers to this dilemma, one possible way forward has been proposed by NCIL (see also Chapter Four for developments in Scotland):

> After considerable consultation with disabled people using Direct Payments ... NCIL proposes that the restrictions on who can be employed by the 'User' are too restrictive. Whilst NCIL would uphold our original stance that immediate relatives living within the same household or separately should be excluded as possible employees (except in exceptional circumstances) other relatives such as cousins, aunts and uncles living in separate accommodation should not be banned. We also wish to see the DoH issue further Guidance on exceptional circumstances. (NCIL, ndb, p 6)

To overcome some of the difficulties of recruiting staff, there is a range of information and advice materials produced by organisations of disabled people as well as a number of support services for disabled people to access. In some areas of the country, direct payment support schemes offer assistance with recruitment, making rooms available for interviews, receiving applications on behalf of disabled employers, typing advertisements, assisting with shortlisting, being present during interviews and so on (see, for example, ILSA, 1998). Peer support mechanisms may also offer disabled people who wish to employ their own PAs the opportunity to meet with other people who have experienced the potential pitfalls of recruitment and discuss possible solutions to common problems. In terms of written information and guidance, the following sources are particularly useful:

- With funding from the Joseph Rowntree Foundation, BCODP (1995) has produced literature on *Controlling your own personal assistance service*. Available via the Internet, this publication provides advice on managing a PA (including drawing up job descriptions, advertising, application forms and interviewing) and includes a sample job description, application form and interview checklist.
- The Disablement Income Group publishes a number of practical guides to recruiting PAs and setting up support schemes (see for example, Dunne with Hoyle, 1992; Simpson with Campbell, 1996). These include practical tips on preparing to recruit, advertising for staff and interviewing.

- The Hampshire Centre for Independent Living (2000) produces a range of advice leaflets (available via the Internet and on paper) on topics such as job descriptions, finding staff and interviewing and choosing staff. These include sample advertisements, interview questions and an application form.
- The Integrated Living Scheme Advice and Support Service (ILSA) (part of the West of England Centre for Integrated Living) produces a practical handbook on self-operated PA schemes, covering a range of financial, legal and administrative issues (ILSA, 1998). Each section of the handbook is colour coded and the section on recruiting staff contains practical examples of job descriptions, application forms, advertisements and sample letters, together with detailed information on relevant legislation and possible places to advertise.

Miscellaneous issues

Receiving direct payments and becoming an employer also raises a number of additional issues, such as:

- arranging emergency cover for workers (ILSA, 1998, pp D1-D4);
- the training and support needs of PAs (Zarb and Nadash, 1994, pp 108-9, Glendinning et al, 2000a);
- the training and support needs of direct payment recipients (Simpson with Campbell, 1996, pp 15-17). Local authority managers would never be asked to recruit and manage staff without adequate training, so why should disabled people be expected to do so?
- managing PAs (BCODP, 1995; Vasey, 2000).

SUMMARY

While many direct payment schemes will already be providing practical advice with regard to these issues, social workers need to be aware of the complexities involved in managing a direct payment so that they can discuss the pros and cons of payments with service users. Recruiting and employing staff can be difficult, and are probably tasks that the vast majority of people (both disabled and non-disabled) would find alien at first. However, with the correct support and information, many disabled people can and do rise to the challenge of becoming employers, organising and monitoring packages of care that meet their needs much more effectively than directly provided services. In many ways, direct payment recipients are acting as their own care managers, and social workers should not be surprised that this is a role that some disabled people are initially unaccustomed to fulfilling. After all, it takes several years of training (both practical and academic) to become a social worker, and disabled people starting to receive direct payments will need varying levels of support as they begin to engage with the practical challenges that managing a payment entails. In seeking to overcome these challenges, a major resource will be the written information produced by organisations of disabled people and the practical experience of other direct payment recipients.

Of course, not everybody will be starting from the same position and different people will have different needs and preferences. For some disabled people, directly provided services or care provided by an agency may offer more security than direct payments and the complexity of managing a payments package may be too much. Others may have extensive experience of receiving payments and may be much better equipped to manage their payments than anybody from the local authority or even from a direct payments support scheme. Most people will probably fall somewhere in between, requiring appropriate assistance to overcome the challenges that direct payments can raise. For these people, accessible information, peer support and an accurate assessment of support needs will be crucial if a direct payments package is to be successful.

TEN

Conclusion: implications for community care

At their best, direct payments have the capacity to transform the lives of disabled people and the work of social services departments, empowering service users and enriching the jobs of social workers. Implemented after a high profile and sustained campaign by organisations of disabled people, direct payments are potentially revolutionary in terms of the opportunities they offer to enhance the choice, control, health and wellbeing of previously marginalised groups of disabled people. In some local authorities, direct payments have been implemented with enthusiasm, benefiting service users, improving satisfaction with care arrangements and leading to greater cost-efficiency. However, this has not always been the case, and many social services departments have been slow to recognise and capitalise on the advantages which direct payments offer. Often, patterns of implementation have been strongly affected by regional variations, with particular areas of the country dragging their heels and hindering progress. In many cases, little consideration has been given to the needs of user groups other than people with physical impairments, and access to payments has often been denied to certain categories of people altogether (despite government guidance). While this is partly due to the wording and focus of legislation and official documentation, it is also the result of discriminatory attitudes and a failure to provide appropriate and accessible information to a range of user groups.

Throughout this book, we have attempted to highlight the strengths and the limitations of direct payment schemes, and the potential advantages and disadvantages of making payments to disabled people in lieu of directly provided services. However, if we are to maximise the positive aspects of direct payments and minimise their potentially negative features, a number of changes will be required, both in social work practice and in official policy.

Practice

The attitude of frontline social workers is crucial to the success or failure of direct payments. Disabled people currently rely on social workers for a great deal of information and cannot be expected to make informed choices about their care arrangements without accurate and accessible advice about the options available to them. Evidence to date suggests that social workers play an important gatekeeping role, and that those people who receive successful payments packages often do so at least in part because of information and support provided by a social worker. At the same time, research also suggests that many practitioners may either be relatively uninformed about direct payments and/or suspicious about the implications of payments for their work. In many cases, fears about an erosion of public services, about losing power and status, about workload implications and about the dangers of creating demands which cannot be met may be hindering the progress of direct payments. In this scenario, it is not disabled people making informed decisions to reject the idea of a direct payments package, but their social workers effectively depriving them of access to direct payments by failing to provide support and information. If direct payments really are to become a central feature of mainstream social services provision, there needs to be much greater emphasis on training for frontline workers and on the provision of accessible information. Although we hope that this book goes some way towards promoting the concept of direct payments, much more work will be required by social work trainers and educators to ensure that staff are appropriately trained, informed and have the right value base for the job they occupy. It will then be down to individual workers to ensure that the people with whom they work:

- are fully informed about the options available to them;
- have the opportunity to think and talk through the advantages and disadvantages of direct payments;
- have sufficient time to make a decision about the type of services they would like to receive;
- have access to peer support so that they can benefit from the experiences of other disabled people.

While this introduction to direct payments does not seek to provide detailed good practice guidance of its own, the authors wish to signpost interested workers towards relevant material produced by organisations of disabled people with considerable experience of the positives and negatives of direct payments. This includes the very detailed but accessible literature cited throughout this book as well as the websites listed in the Appendix. It is our firm belief that direct payments offer practitioners a new and extremely exciting way of working, empowering service users to be more in control of their own lives. Whether or not individual social workers are prepared to accept this challenge is ultimately down to them.

Policy

In addition to changes in the training and attitudes of frontline workers, a number of policy measures will be required to promote direct payments, removing existing limitations while at the same time retaining the many advantages that existing payment packages have to offer. In order to extend direct payments to a greater number of people and to a wider range of user groups, policy makers need to reconsider the emphasis on being 'willing and able', exploring the potential of new ways of working to safeguard the rights of people with profound learning difficulties. Greater consideration should also be given to the barriers faced by users other than those with physical impairments and to people who are gay/lesbian or from minority ethnic groups. At the same time, policy makers must re-examine issues such as the level of payments that are being made, sources of funding for establishing direct payment schemes and providing peer support, the employment of relatives, the health and social care divide, charging policies, accountability arrangements and cost ceilings.

Overall, the overriding message from this introduction to direct payments is the central role that has been played by disabled people in campaigning for direct payments and making payment schemes work. Ultimately, direct payments are not an end in themselves, but simply a means to an end (that is, independent living). For direct payments to be truly successful and to become part of mainstream social services provision, social work policy and practice will need to be consistent with the goals of the Independent Living Movement and be guided by the considerable expertise of disabled people.

Bibliography

Abbott, P. (2000) 'Gender', in G. Payne (ed) *Social divisions*, Basingstoke: Macmillan.

Adams, I. (1998) *Ideology and politics in Britain today*, Manchester: Manchester University Press.

Age Concern (1998) 'Extend direct payments to over 65s', *Care Plan*, vol 5, no 2, pp 14-16.

Age Concern (2000) *Direct payments from social services*, Factsheet 24, London: Age Concern England.

Alcock, P. (1996) *Social policy in Britain: Themes and issues*, Basingstoke: Macmillan.

Andrisani, P. and Nestel, G. (1976) 'Internal–external control as contributor to and outcome of work experience', *Journal of Applied Psychology*, vol 61, no 2, pp 156-65.

Arber, S. and Ginn, J. (1995a) 'Gender differences in informal caring', *Health and Social Care in the Community*, vol 3, no 1, pp 19-31.

Arber, S. and Ginn, J. (1995b) 'Gender differences in the relationship between paid employment and informal care', *Work, Employment & Society*, vol 9, no 3, pp 445-71.

Aspis, S. (1996a) 'Direct Payments Bill: good in principle but limited in scope', *Community Living*, January, pp 4-5.

Aspis, S. (1996b) 'How can people always denied choices express a preference', *Community Living*, vol 10, no 2, pp 3-4.

Aspis, S. (1998) *Users' ability to manage direct payments*, London: Changing Perspectives/NCIL.

Audit Commission (1986) *Making a reality of community care*, London: HMSO.

Audit Commission (1999) *The price is right? Charges for council services*, London: Audit Commission.

Auld, F. (1999) *Community Care (Direct Payments) Act 1996: Analysis of responses to local authority questionnaire on implementation – England*, London: DoH.

Bailey, R. (2000) 'Don't forget the police', *Personal Assistants Users' Newsletter*, October, pp 9-10.

Balloch, S., McLean, J. and Fisher, M. (eds) (1999) *Social services: Working under pressure*, Bristol: The Policy Press.

Barnes, C. (ed) (1993) *Making our own choices: Independent living, personal assistance and disabled people*, Belper: BCODP.

Barnes, C. (1995) *From national to local: An evaluation of the effectiveness of national disablement information providers' information services to local disablement information providers*, London: BCODP.

Barnes, C. (1997) *Older people's perceptions of direct payments and self-operated support schemes*, Leeds: BCODP Research Unit.

Barnes, M. (1997) *Care, communities and citizens*, London: Longman.

Barnes, M. and Walker, A. (1996) 'Consumerism versus empowerment: a principled approach to the involvement of older service users', *Policy & Politics*, vol 24, no 4, pp 375-94.

Barnett, H. (1918) *Canon Barnett: His life, work and friends – Volume One*, London: John Murray.

Barret, G. and Hudson, M. (1997) 'Changes in district nursing workload', *Journal of Community Nursing*, vol 11, no 3, pp 4-8.

Beardshaw, V. (1988) *Last on the list: Community services for people with physical disabilities*, London: King's Fund.

Becker, S. (1997) *Responding to poverty: The politics of cash and care*, Basingstoke: Macmillan.

Becker, S. and MacPherson, S. (eds) (1988) *Public issues, private pain: Poverty, social work and social policy*, London: Insight/Carematters Books.

Begum, N. (1993) 'Independent living, personal assistance and disabled women', in C. Barnes (ed) *Making our own choices: Independent living, personal assistance and disabled people*, Belper: BCODP.

Beresford, P. (1996) 'Meet the diversity of need', *Care Plan*, vol 2, no 4, p 14.

Bewley, C. (1998) *Choice and control: Decision-making and people with learning difficulties*, London: Values Into Action.

Bewley, C. (2000a) 'Care managers can be champions for direct payments', *Care Plan*, vol 6, no 4, pp 13-16.

Bewley, C. (2000b) 'Tribunal ruling has no legal relevance for direct payments', *Community Living*, vol 13, no 3, p 3.

Bewley, C. (2000c) 'Vital lessons to be learned from the South Lanarkshire ruling', *Community Living*, vol 13, no 4, pp 9-11.

Bignall, T. and Butt, J. (2000) *Between ambition and achievement: Young black disabled people's views and experiences of independence and independent living*, Bristol/York: The Policy Press/Joseph Rowntree Foundation.

Bond, H. (1996) 'State of independence', *Community Care*, 4-10 April, pp 20-1.

Bosanquet, H. (1914) *Social work in London 1869-1912: A history of the Charity Organisation Society*, London: John Murray.

Brandon, D. (1998) 'What is direct payment?', *Breakthrough*, vol 2, no 3, pp 25-6.

Brandon, D., Maglajlic, R. and Given, D. (2000) 'The information deficit hinders progress', *Care Plan*, vol 6, no 4, pp 17-20.

Brindle, D. (2000) 'Ticket to independence', *Guardian Society*, 11 October.

BCODP (ed) (1995) *Controlling your own personal assistance services* (www.independentliving.org/ENIL/ENILBCODPPaySchemes.html: accessed 30 January 2001).

Browne, L. (1990) *Survey of local authorities direct payments*, London: RADAR.

Burgess, P. (1994) 'Welfare rights,' in C. Hanvey and T. Philpot (eds) *Practising social work*, London: Routledge.

Burrows, G. (2001) 'Charities criticise draft home care standards', *Community Care*, 21-27 June, p 3.

Butt, J. and Box, L. (1997) *Supportive services, effective strategies: The views of black-led organisations and social care agencies on the future of social care for black communities*, London: Race Equalities Unit.

Butt, J., Bignall, T. and Stone, E. (eds) (2000) *Directing support: Report from a workshop on direct payments and black and minority ethnic disabled people*, York: Joseph Rowntree Foundation.

Campbell, J. (nd) 'Promoting personal assistance to enable independent living', Social Services Conference, 29 October, London: NCIL.

Campbell, J. (1996) 'Implementing direct payments: towards the next millennium', National Institute of Social Work Conference, 12 November.

Care Development Group (2001) *Fair care for older people*, Edinburgh: Scottish Executive.

Care Plan (1996a) 'Direct payments – an idea whose time has come', *Care Plan*, vol 2, no 4, p 8.

Care Plan (1996b) 'The empowerment of money', *Care Plan*, vol 2, no 3, pp 12-13.

Care Plan (1997) 'Money for services – let partnerships prevail', *Care Plan*, vol 3, no 4, pp 29-30.

Carmichael, F. and Charles, S. (1998) 'The labour market costs of community care', *Journal of Health Economics*, vol 17, no 6, pp 747-65.

Chinn, C. (1995) *Poverty amidst prosperity: The urban poor in England, 1834-1914*, Manchester: Manchester University Press.

CIPFA (Chartered Institute of Public Finance and Accountancy) (1998) *Community care direct payments: Accounting and financial management guidelines*, London: CIPFA.

Clark, H. and Spafford, J. (2001a) *Piloting choice and control for older people: An evaluation*, Joseph Rowntree Foundation Findings 431, York: Joseph Rowntree Foundation.

Clark, H. and Spafford, J. (2001b) *Piloting choice and control for older people: An evaluation*, Bristol: The Policy Press.

Clark, H., Dyer, S. and Horwood, J. (1998) *That bit of help: The high value of low level preventative services for older people*, Bristol/York: The Policy Press/Joseph Rowntree Foundation.

Clements, T. (1996) 'Direct payments: are they all good news?', *Community Living*, vol 10, no 2, p 10.

Collins, J. (1996) 'A little help from a friend to reach the 'unachievable', *Care Plan*, vol 2, no 4, p 13.

Collins, J. (1997) 'Direct payments are not a mystery', *Care Plan*, vol 4, no 1, pp 18-20.

Community Care (1997) 'Direct payments in doubt', *Community Care*, 13-19 March, p 6.

Community Care (1999) 'Local authorities are liable for personal assistants', *Community Care*, 5-11 August, p 4.

Community Living (1999a) '"Direct payments – a person's impairment should not make them ineligible", says guide', *Community Living*, vol 12, no 3, p 2.

Community Living (1999b) 'How to get a direct payments scheme', *Community Living*, vol 13, no 1, p 21.

Coolen, J. and Weekers, S. (1998) 'Long-term care in the Netherlands: public funding and private provision within a universalistic welfare state', in C. Glendinning (ed) *Rights and realities: Comparing new developments in long-term care for older people*, Bristol: The Policy Press.

Craig, G. (1992) *Cash or care: A question of choice? Cash, community care and user participation*, York: Social Policy Research Unit, University of York.

D'Abouville, E. (1995) *Commissioning independent living: A guide to developing personal assistance schemes and support services*, London: King's Fund.

Davis, A. (1996) 'Women and the personal social services', in C. Hallett (ed) *Women and social policy*, London: Harvester Wheatsheaf.

Davis, A. and Stephenson, D. (1999) 'Working with poor communities: social and community work in the UK – one hundred years of change and continuity', Unpublished paper presented at Association House, 20 October, Chicago.

Davis, A. and Wainwright, S. (1996) 'Poverty work and the mental health services', *Breakthrough*, vol 1, no 1, pp 47-55.

Davis, A., Ellis, K. and Rummery, K. (1997) *Access to assessment: Perspectives of practitioners, disabled people and carers*, Bristol: The Policy Press.

Dawson, C. (1995) *Report of the Independent Living Project (Norfolk)*, Cambridge: Daniels Publications/Joseph Rowntree Foundation.

Dawson, C. (2000) *Independent successes: Implementing direct payments*, York: Joseph Rowntree Foundation.

Dawson, C. and McDonald, A. (2000) 'Assessing mental capacity – a checklist for social workers', *Practice*, vol 12, no 2, pp 5-20.

DHSSPS (Department of Health, Social Services and Public Safety (1997) *Personal Social Services (Direct Payments) (Northern Ireland) Order 1996: Guidance for boards and trusts*, Belfast: DHSSPS.

DHSSPS (2000a) *A guide to receiving direct payments*, Belfast: The Stationery Office.

DHSSPS (2000b) *Personal Social Services (Direct Payments) (Northern Ireland) Order 1996: Guidance for boards and trusts*, Belfast: DHSSPH.

Dickens, C. (1867) *Oliver Twist*, London: Chapman and Hall.

Disablement Income Group (1996) *Personal assistance support schemes and the introduction of direct payments: A report and recommendations*, London: Disablement Income Group.

DoH (Department of Health) (1989) *Caring for people: Community care in the next decade and beyond*, London: HMSO.

DoH (1990) *Community care in the next decade and beyond: Policy guidance*, London: DoH.

DoH (1994) 'Virginia Bottomley gives direct payments to disabled people the go ahead', 24 November, Press Release 94/537, London: DoH.

DoH (1997a) *Community Care (Direct Payments) Act 1996: Policy and practice guidance*, London: DoH.

DoH (1997b) *Direct Payments Act: Presentation materials*, London: DoH.

DoH (1998a) *Modernising social services: Promoting independence, improving protection, raising standards*, London: The Stationery Office.

DoH (1998b) *A guide to receiving direct payments*, London: DoH.

DoH (1998c) 'Independence pays: Community Care (Direct Payments) Act 1996', with Subtitles, information video, London: DoH.

DoH (1998d) *Partnership in action: New opportunities for joint working between health and social services – A discussion document*, London: DoH.

DoH (1999) 'Direct payments: Cash for services', information video, London: DoH.

DoH (2000a) *Community Care (Direct Payments) Act 1996: Policy and practice guidance* (2nd edn), London: DoH.

DoH (2000b) *An easy guide to direct payments*, London: DoH.

DoH (2000c) *Explanatory notes to Carers and Disabled Children Act 2000*, London: The Stationery Office.

DoH (2000d) *The NHS Plan: A plan for investment, a plan for reform*, London: The Stationery Office.

DoH (2000e) *The NHS Plan: The government's response to the Royal Commission on Long-Term Care*, London: The Stationery Office.

DoH (2000f) *Caring about carers: A national strategy for carers* (2nd edn), London: DoH.

DoH (2001a) *Carers and Disabled Children Act 2000: Carers and people with parental responsibility for disabled children – Practice guidance*, London: DoH.

DoH (2001b) *Carers and Disabled Children Act 2000: Carers and people with parental responsibility for disabled children – Policy guidance*, London: DoH.

DoH (2001c) *Carers and Disabled Children Act 2000: Direct payments for young disabled people – Policy guidance and practice guidance*, London: DoH.

DoH (2001d) *A practitioner's guide to carers' assessments under the Carers and Disabled Children Act 2000*, London: DoH.

DoH (2001e) *Explanatory notes to Health and Social Care Act 2001* (www.legislation.hmso.gov.uk/acts/en/2001en15.htm: accessed 19 June 2001).

DoH (2001f) *Valuing people: A new strategy for learning disability for the 21st century*, London: DoH.

DoH (2001g) *Fairer charging policies for home care and other non-residential social services: A consultation paper*, London: DoH.

DoH (2001h) *Fairer charging policies for home care and other non-residential social services: Draft guidance*, London: DoH.

DoH/Scottish Office/Welsh Office/Northern Ireland Office (1996) *Community Care (Direct Payments) Bill: Consultation paper*, London: DoH.

DoH/SSI (Social Services Inspectorate) (1991) *Care management and assessment: Practitioners' guide*, London: HMSO.

DoH/SSI (1996) *Progressing services with physically disabled people: Report on inspections of community services for physically disabled people*, London: DoH.

DoH/SSI (1997) *Inspection of community care services for black and minority ethnic older people: Birmingham*, Nottingham: Central Inspection Group, SSI.

DoH/SSI (1999a) *Inspection of independent living arrangements for younger disabled people: Poole Borough Council*, Bristol: South and West Inspection Group, SSI.

DoH/SSI (1999b) *Inspection of independent living arrangements for younger disabled people: Middlesbrough Borough Council*, Gateshead: North East Inspection Group, SSI.

DoH/SSI (1999c) *Inspection of independent living arrangements for younger disabled people: County of Herefordshire District Council*, Bristol: South and West Inspection Group, SSI.

DoH/SSI (1999d) *Inspection of independent living arrangements for younger disabled people: Oxfordshire County Council*, Bristol: South and West Inspection Group, SSI.

DoH/SSI (1999e) *Inspection of independent living arrangements for younger disabled people: Lincolnshire County Council*, Nottingham: East Inspection Group, SSI.

DoH/SSI (1999f) *Inspection of independent living arrangements for younger disabled people: London Borough of Enfield*, London: London Inspection Group, SSI.

DoH/SSI (1999g) *Inspection of independent living arrangements for younger disabled people: The City of Westminster*, London: London Inspection Group, SSI.

DoH/SSI (1999h) *Inspection of independent living arrangements for younger disabled people: Stockport MBC*, Manchester: North West Inspection Group, SSI.

DoH/SSI (1999i) *Inspection of independent living arrangements for younger disabled people: Metropolitan Borough of Calderdale*, Gateshead: North East Inspection Group, SSI.

DoH/SSI (1999j) *Inspection of independent living arrangements for younger disabled people: Brighton and Hove*, London: South Inspection Group, SSI.

Drew, E. (1995) 'Employment prospects of carers of dependent adults', *Health and Social Care in the Community*, vol 3, no 5, pp 325-31.

Dunne, M. with Hoyle, J. (1992) *Recruiting and employing a personal care worker*, London: Disablement Income Group.

Dunnicliff, J. (1999) *Funding for personal assistance support services: The key to making personal assistance schemes work*, London: NCIL.

Edsall, N.C. (1971) *The anti-Poor Law movement, 1834-1844*, Manchester: Manchester University Press.

Elkington, G. (1996) 'Exceptions to the rule', *Care Plan*, vol 2, no 4, p 12.

Ellis, K., Davis, A. and Rummery, K. (1999) 'Needs assessment, street-level bureaucracy and the new community care', *Social Policy and Administration*, vol 33, no 3, pp 262-80.

Englander, D. (1998) *Poverty and Poor Law reform in 19th century Britain, 1834-1914: From Chadwick to Booth*, London: Longman.

ENIL (European Network on Independent Living) (1997) *Training on direct payments for personal assistance*, Report from the ENIL Seminar, Berlin, 1-4 May (www.independentliving.org/ENIL/ENILReport9705.htm: accessed 01 March 2001).

ENIL (1999) *About ENIL* (www.independentliving.org/ENIL/: accessed 30 January 2001).

European Union (2000) *Council Directive 2000/78/EC of 27 November 2000 establishing a General Framework for Equal Treatment in Employment and Occupation* (http://europa.eu.int/eur-lex/en/lif/dat/2000/en_300L0078.html: accessed 21 January 2002).

Evans, J. (1993) 'The role of centres of independent/integrated living and networks of disabled people', in C. Barnes (ed) *Making our own choices: Independent living, personal assistance and disabled people*, Belper: BCODP.

Evans, J. (2000) 'Direct payments in the United Kingdom', Presentation at the International Conference on Self-Determination and Individualised Funding, Seattle, 29-31 July.

Evans, J. and Hasler, F. (1996) 'Direct Payments Campaign in the UK', Presentation for the European Network on Independent Living Seminar, Stockholm, 9-11 June.

Evers, A., Pijl, M. and Ungerson, C. (eds) (1994) *Payments for care: A comparative overview*, Aldershot: Avebury.

Francis, R. (2001) 'Direct payments: helping service users become service consumers', *Link Up*, Winter, pp 4-8.

Fraser, D. (1984) *The evolution of the British welfare state* (2nd edn), Basingstoke: Macmillan.

Friedman, M. (1962) *Capitalism and freedom*, Chicago, IL: University of Chicago Press.

Fruin, D. (1998) *Moving into the mainstream: The report of a national inspection of services for adults with learning disabilities*, London: DoH.

Fruin, D. (2000) *New directions for independent living*, London: DoH.

Fryer, R. (1998) *Signposts to services: Inspection of social services information to the public*, London: DoH.

Gardner, A. (1999) *Making direct payments a reality for people with learning difficulties*, Whalley: North West Training and Development Team.

George, M. (1994a) 'Flexible choices', *Community Care*, 24-30 November, pp 14-15.

George, M. (1994b) 'Paying direct', *Community Care*, 25-31 August, pp 14-15.

George, M. (1996) 'Cash on the nail', *Community Care*, 17-23 October, pp 24-5.

George, M. (2001) 'Our way or no way', *Community Care*, 12-18 July, pp 32-3.

Ginn, J. and Sandell, J. (1997), 'Balancing home and employment: stress reported by social services staff', *Work, Employment & Society*, vol 11, no 3, pp 413-34.

Glasby, J. (1999) *Poverty and opportunity: 100 years of the Birmingham Settlement*, Studley: Brewin Books.

Glasby, J. (2000a) 'Mixed blessings: is the NHS Plan revolutionary?', *British Journal of Nursing*, vol 18, p 9.

Glasby, J. (2000b) 'Bringing down the Berlin Wall', *Nursing Older People*, vol 12, no 7, p 6.

Glasby, J. (2001a) 'Bringing down the "Berlin Wall": the health and social care divide', *British Journal of Social Work*, (forthcoming).

Glasby, J. (2001b) 'A direct route for cash', *Community Care*, 28 January, pp 25-31.

Glasby, J. and Glasby, J. (1999) *Paying for social services: Social services and local government finance*, Birmingham: PEPAR Publications.

Glasby, J. and Littlechild, R. (2000a) 'Fighting fires? Emergency hospital admission and the concept of prevention', *Journal of Management in Medicine*, vol 14, no 2, pp 109-18.

Glasby, J. and Littlechild, R. (2000b) *The health and social care divide: The experiences of older people*, Birmingham: PEPAR Publications.

Glasby, J. and Littlechild, R. (2000c) 'Falling into the chasm', *Nursing Older People*, vol 12, no 8, pp 32-3.

Glendinning, C., Haliwell, S., Jacobs, S., Rummery, K. and Tyrer, J. (2000a) *Buying independence: Using direct payments to integrate health and social services*, Bristol: The Policy Press.

Glendinning, C., Haliwell, S., Jacobs, S., Rummery, K. and Tyrer, J. (2000b) 'Bridging the gap: using direct payments to purchase integrated care', *Health and Social Care in the Community*, vol 8, no 3, pp 192-200.

Glendinning, C., Haliwell, S., Jacobs, S., Rummery, K. and Tyrer, J. (2000c) 'New kinds of care, new kinds of relationships: how purchasing services affects relationships in giving and receiving personal assistance', *Health and Social Care in the Community*, vol 8, no 3, pp 201-11.

Goodinge, S. (2000) *A jigsaw of services: Inspection of services to support disabled adults in their parenting role*, London: DoH.

Goodman, C. (1986) 'Research on the informal carer: a selected literature review', *Journal of Advanced Nursing*, vol 11, pp 705-12.

Greenwood, W. (1969) *Love on the dole*, Harmondsworth: Penguin.

Grimshaw, J. and Fletcher, S. (nd) *Direct payments: People with HIV – The way forward*, London: National AIDS Trust/NCIL.

Hallett, C. (ed) (1989) *Women and social services departments*, London: Harvester Wheatsheaf.

Halloran, J. (ed) (1998) *Towards a people's Europe: A report on the development of direct payments in 10 member states of the European Union*, Vienna: European Social Network.

Hampshire Centre for Independent Living (2000) *Advice sheets* (www.hants.gov.uk/socservs/directpayments/dpadvicesheets.htm: accessed 30 January 2001).

Hancock, R. and Jarvis, C. (1995) 'Care free? The after effects of being a carer', *Reviews in Clinical Gerontology*, vol 5, no 3, pp 245-6.

Hasler, F. (1997) 'Living is about more than bed and breakfast', *Health Matters*, vol 32, pp 12-13.

Hasler, F. (1999) 'Exercising the right to freedom of choice', *Professional Social Work*, June, pp 6-7.

Hasler, F. (2000) 'What is direct payments', in J. Butt, T. Bignall and E. Stone (eds) *Directing support: Report from a workshop on direct payments and black and minority ethnic disabled people*, York: Joseph Rowntree Foundation.

Hasler, F. and Zarb, G. (2000) *Direct payments and older people*, Social Services Research Group Annual Workshop, 13 April.

Hasler, F., Campbell, J. and Zarb, G. (1999) *Direct routes to independence: A guide to local authority implementation and management of direct payments*, London: Policy Studies Institute.

Hasler, F., Zarb, G. and Campbell, J. (1998) *Key issues for local authority implementation of direct payments* (first published 1998, revised 1999) (www.psi.org.uk/publications/DISAB/key%20issues.htm: accessed 18 January 2001).

Hatchett, W. (1991) 'Cash on delivery?', *Community Care*, 30 May, pp 14-15.

Hayek, F. (1944) *The road to serfdom*, London: Routledge and Kegan Paul.

Henderson, E. and Bewley, C. (2000) *Too little, too slowly: Report on direct payments for people with learning difficulties in Scotland*, London: Values Into Action.

Henwood, M. (1998) *Ignored and invisible? Carers' experience of the NHS*, London: Carers National Association.

Henwood, M. and Wistow, G. (1993) *Hospital discharge and community care: Early days*, Leeds: Nuffield Institute for Health.

Henwood, M., Hardy, B., Hudson, B. and Wistow, G. (1997) *Inter-agency collaboration: Hospital discharge and continuing care sub-study*, Leeds: Nuffield Institute for Health Community Care Division.

Heslop, P. (2001) 'Direct payments for people with mental health support needs', *The Advocate*, May, pp 8-9.

Hill, M. (ed) (2000) *Local authority social services: An introduction*, Oxford: Blackwell.

Hirst, J. (1997) 'Direct benefit?', *Community Care*, 1 May, pp 10-11.

Hoffmann, R. and Mitchell, A. (1998) 'Caregiver burden: historical development', *Nursing Forum*, vol 33, no 4, pp 5-11.

Holman, A. (1995) 'Sample trust deed', London: Values into Action.

Holman, A. (1996) 'VIA fights to amend clause on direct payments', *Community Living*, vol 10, no 2, p 2.

Holman, A. (1998a) *Funding freedom: Direct payments for people with learning difficulties*, Values Into Action leaflet and tape, London: Values Into Action.

Holman, A. (1998b) *Make your move: A video guide to independent living for all people with learning difficulties*, London: Values Into Action.

Holman, A. and Bewley, C. (1999) *Funding freedom 2000: People with learning difficulties using direct payments*, London: Values into Action.

Holman, A. and Collins, J. (1997) *Funding freedom: Direct payments for people with learning difficulties*, London: Values into Action.

House of Commons Health Committee (1993) *Community care: The way forward – Volume I* (Sixth Report), London: HMSO.

Howarth, J., Graham, M. and Townsley, R. (2000) 'Head, heart and hands', *Community Living*, April/May, pp 12-13.

Howe, D. (1986) 'The segregation of women and their work in the personal social services, *Critical Social Policy*, vol 5, no 3, pp 21-35.

HSE (Health and Safety Executive) (1995) *Health and safety regulations: A short guide*, London: HSE.

HSE (2000) *Getting to grips with manual handling: A short guide for employers*, London: HSE.

Hudson, B. (1988) 'Doomed from the start?', *Health Service Journal*, 23 June, pp 708-9.

Hudson, B. (1993) 'The Icarus effect', *Health Service Journal*, 18 November, pp 27-9.

Hudson, B. (1994) 'Independent living for people in Britain: too successful by half? The case of the Independent Living Fund', *Critical Social Policy*, vol 40, pp 88-96.

Hudson, B. (2000) 'Inter-agency collaboration: a sceptical view', in A. Brechin, H. Brown and M.A. Eby (eds) *Critical practice in health and social care*, London: Sage Publications, in association with the Open University.

Hudson, B., Hardy, B., Henwood, M. and Wistow, G. (1997) *Inter-agency collaboration: Final report*, Leeds: Nuffield Institute for Health Community Care Division.

Hunter, M. (1999) 'Case threatens direct payments', *Community Care*, 12-18 August, pp 10-11.

(ILF) Independent Living Fund (2000) *Guidance notes for the 93 Fund and Extension Fund*, Nottingham: Independent Living Fund.

ILSA (Independent Living Scheme Advice and Support Service) (1998) *Personal assistant employer's handbook*, Bristol: West of England Centre for Integrated Living.

Irish, H. (1998) 'Direct payments', *Breakthrough*, vol 2, no 3, pp 27-32.

Jones, G. (1989) Women in social care: the invisible army', in C. Hallett (ed) *Women and social services departments*, London: Harvester Wheatsheaf.

Jones, R. (2000) *Getting going on direct payments*, Trowbridge: Wiltshire Social Services, on behalf of the Association of Directors of Social Services.

Jordan, B. (1974) *Poor parents: Social policy and the 'cycle of deprivation'*, London: Routledge and Kegan Paul.

Kempson, E. (1995) *Money and debt counselling*, London: Policy Studies Institute.

Kestenbaum, A. (1993a) *Making community care a reality: The Independent Living Fund, 1988-1993*, London: RADAR.

Kestenbaum, A. (1993b) *Cash for care: A report on the experience of Independent Living Fund clients* (2nd edn), London: RADAR/Disablement Income Group.

Kestenbaum, A. (1996) 'The state of independence', *Community Care*, 22-28 February, pp 32-3.

Kestenbaum, A. (1998) *Work, rest and pay: The deal for personal assistance users*, York: York Publishing Services.

Kestenbaum, A. (1999) *What price independence? Independent living and people with high support needs*, Bristol/York: The Policy Press/Joseph Rowntree Foundation.

Killin, D. (1993) 'Independent living, personal assistance, disabled lesbians and gay men', in C. Barnes (ed) *Making our own choices: Independent living, personal assistance and disabled people*, Belper: BCODP.

Kobasa, S. (1979) 'Stressful life events, personality and health: an inquiry into hardiness', *Journal of Personality and Social Psychology*, vol 37, no 1, pp 1-11.

Lakey, J. (1994) *Caring about independence: Disabled people and the Independent Living Fund*, London: Policy Studies Institute.

Leece, J. (2000) 'It's a matter of choice: making direct payments work in Staffordshire', *Practice*, vol 12, no 4, pp 37-48.

Leedham, I. (1996) 'Contracting with 'ordinary people' ('helpers'): approaches and issues', *CCMP*, vol 4, no 2, pp 41-7.

Lewis, J. (1995) *The voluntary sector, the state and social work in Britain*, Aldershot: Edward Elgar.

Lewis, J. (1996) 'What does contracting do to voluntary agencies?', in D. Billis and M. Harris (eds) *Voluntary agencies: Challenges of organisations and management*, Basingstoke: Macmillan.

Lipsky, M. (1980) *Street-level bureaucracy: Dilemmas of the individual in public services*, New York, NY: Russell Sage Foundation.

Luckhurst, L. (2000) 'Survivors explore direct payments', *Personal Assistants Users' Newsletter*, August, pp 11-12.

Luckhurst, L. (2001) 'What does the term "direct payments" mean to you?', *The Advocate*, May, pp 6-7.

McCurry, P. (1999) 'The direct route', *Community Care*, 9-15 September, pp 20-1.

Macfarlane, A. (1990) 'The right to make choices', *Community Care*, 1 November, pp 14-15.

McKay, S. and Rowlingson, K. (1999) *Social security in Britain*, Basingstoke: Macmillan.

McLaughlin, E. and Ritchie, J. (1994) 'Legacies of caring: the experiences and circumstances of ex-carers', *Health and Social Care in the Community*, vol 2, no 4, pp 241-53.

Maglajlic, R. (1999) 'The silent treatment', *Openmind*, September/October, pp 12-13.

Maglajlic, R., Brandon, D. and Given, D. (2000) 'Making direct payments a choice: a report on the research findings', *Disability & Society*, vol 15, no 1, pp 99-113.

Maglajlic, R., Bryant, M., Brandon, D. and Given, D. (1998) 'Direct payments in mental health – a research report', *Breakthrough*, vol 2, no 3, pp 33-43.

Mandelstam, M. (1999) *Community care practice and the law* (2nd edn), London: Jessica Kingsley.

Means, R. and Smith, R. (1998a) *Community care: Policy and practice* (2nd edn), Basingstoke: Macmillan.

Means, R. and Smith, R. (1998b) *From Poor Law to community care: The development of welfare services for elderly people, 1939-1971* (2nd edn), Bristol: The Policy Press.

Morris, J. (1993a) *Independent lives: Community care and disabled people*, Basingstoke: Macmillan.

Morris, J. (1993b) 'Advocating true reform', *Community Care*, 4 February, pp 16-17.

Morris, J. (1993c) *Community care or independent living?*, York: Joseph Rowntree Foundation.

Morris, J. (1995) 'How to get money to pay for personal assistance and have control over how its spent', in BCODP (ed) *Controlling your own personal assistance services* (www.independent living.org/ ENILBCODPPaySchemes.html: accessed 30 January 2001).

Morris, J. (1997) 'Care or empowerment? A disability rights perspective', *Social Policy and Administration*, vol 31, no 1, pp 54-60.

Murray, C. (1984) *Losing ground: American social policy 1950-1980*, New York, NY: Basic Books.

National Assembly for Wales (1997) *Community Care (Direct Payments) Act 1996: Policy and practice guidance*, Cardiff: National Assembly for Wales.

National Assembly for Wales (2000) *Community Care (Direct Payments) Act 1996: Policy and practice guidance*, Cardiff: National Assembly for Wales.

NCIL (National Centre for Independent Living) (nda) 'Promoting personal assistance to enable independent living', Unpublished information sheet, London: NCIL.

NCIL (ndb) *Community Care (Direct Payments) Act 1996 government review: Response by the British Council of Disabled People's National Centre for Independent Living*, London, NCIL.

NCIL (ndc) *Direct payments for mental health users/survivors* (www.ncil.org.uk/ dpays_mh_users.asp: accessed 18 October 2001).

NCIL (ndd) *Response to consultation on CIPFA draft guidance on direct payments*, London: NCIL.

NCIL (1988) *Employing personal assistants: The key facts about their terms and conditions of employment*, London: NCIL.

NCIL (1999) *Government White Paper: Modernising social services – Response by the British Council of Disabled People's National Centre for Independent Living*, London: NCIL.

NCIL (2000a) *NCIL Briefing on the Carers and Disabled Children Bill*, London: NCIL.

NCIL (2000b) *Personal assistance support schemes: Complete list – June-July 2000*, London: NCIL.

Novak, T. (1988) *Poverty and the state: An historical sociology*, Buckingham: Open University Press.

NWTDT (North West Training and Development Team) (2000a) 'Making direct payments happen for people with learning difficulties', Unpublished leaflet, Whalley: NWTDT.

NWTDT (2000b) 'Access to direct payments for people with learning difficulties', Unpublished leaflet, Whalley: NWTDT.

Oliver, M. (1990) *The politics of disablement*, Basingstoke: Macmillan.

Oliver, M. (1996) *Understanding disability: From theory to practice*, Basingstoke: Macmillan.

Oliver, M. and Sapey, B. (1999) *Social work with disabled people* (2nd edn), Basingstoke: Macmillan.

Oliver, M. and Zarb, G. (1992) *Greenwich personal assistance schemes: Second year evaluation*, London: Greenwich Association of Disabled People.

Pearson, C. (2000) 'Money talks? Competing discourses in the role of direct payments', *Critical Social Policy*, vol 20, no 4, pp 459-77.

Pierce, A. (1996) 'Ministers strive to quell revolt over cash for disabled', *The Times*, 7 June.

Pijl, M. (1997) 'Quality of care: on whose terms?', in A. Evers, R. Haverinen, K. Leichsenring and G. Wistow (eds) *Developing quality in personal social services: Concepts, cases and comments*, Aldershot: Ashgate.

Pijl, M. (2000) 'Home care allowances: good for many but not for all', *Practice*, vol 12, no 2, pp 55-65.

Project 81 (nd) *Project 81 – One step up*, Petersfield: HCIL Papers.

Ratzka, A. (nd) 'What is independent living?', Unpublished information sheet, London: NCIL.

Rees, S. (1978) *Social work face to face*, London: Edward Arnold.

Revans, L. (2000) 'Payments reform stalls', *Community Care*, 28 September-4 October, p 12.

Rickford, F. (1996) 'Home free', *Community Care*, 18-24 January, pp 20-1.

Riley, C. (1999) 'Directly involved? A study of direct payments', Unpublished Masters dissertation, Department of Social Policy and Social Work, University of Birmingham.

Rooff, M. (1972) *One hundred years of family social work: A study of the family welfare society 1868-1969*, London: Michael Joseph.

Rose, M.E. (1988) *The relief of poverty, 1834-1914* (2nd edn), Basingstoke: Macmillan.

Routledge, M. and Sanderson, H. (2000) *Work in progress: Implementing person centred planning in Oldham*, Whalley: NWTDT.

Royal Commission on Long Term Care (1999) *With respect to old age: Long term care – Rights and responsibilities*, London: The Stationery Office.

Ryan, T. and Holman, A. (1998a) *Able and willing? Supporting people with learning difficulties to use direct payments*, London: Values Into Action.

Ryan, T. and Holman, A. (1998b) 'Questions of control and consent', *Care Plan*, vol 5, no 2, pp 10-14.

Ryan, T. and Holman, A. (1998c) *Pointers to control: People with learning difficulties using direct payments*, London: Values Into Action.

Sanderson, H. and Kilbane, J. (1999) *Person centred planning – A resource guide*, Whalley: NWTDT.

Satyamurti, C. (1981) *Occupational survival*, Oxford: Blackwell.

Schunk, M. (1998) 'The social insurance model of care for older people in Germany', in C. Glendinning (ed) *Rights and realities: Comparing new developments in long-term care for older people*, Bristol: The Policy Press.

Scottish Executive (2000) 'Direct payments extended', Scottish Executive press release SE1749/2000, 15/06/2000, Edinburgh: Scottish Executive.

Scottish Executive (2001) 'Chisholm announces £530,000 to promote direct payments', Scottish Executive press release SE0940/2001, 06/04/2001, Edinburgh: Scottish Executive.

Scottish Executive Central Research Unit (2001) *Direct payments for mental health service users: Research specification*, Edinburgh: Scottish Executive Central Research Unit.

Scottish Office (1997) *Community Care (Direct Payments) Act 1996: Policy and practice guidance*, Edinburgh: Scottish Office Social Work Services Group.

Scottish Office (2000) *Community Care (Direct Payments) Act 1996: Policy and practice guidance*, Edinburgh: Scottish Office Social Work Services Group.

Seligman, M.E.P. (1975) *Helplessness: On depression, development and death*, San Francisco, CA: W.H. Freeman.

Shearer, A. (1984) 'Independence is the name of the game', *Voluntary Action*, vol 2, no 3, pp 10-11.

Simpson, F. with Campbell, J. (1996) *Facilitating and supporting independent living: A guide to setting up a personal assistance support scheme*, London: Disablement Income Group.

Taylor, R. (1994) 'Putting the cash upfront', *ADSS News*, November, pp 16-17.

Taylor, R. (1995) *Community Care (Direct Payments) Bill: Briefing paper*, Kingston-upon-Thames: ADSS Disabilities Committee.

Taylor, R. (1996a) 'Independent living and direct payments', Speech delivered to the ADSS Spring Conference, Cambridge, April.

Taylor, R. (1996b) 'A coherent policy for direct payments', *ADSS News*, vol 5, no 4, p 20.

Taylor, R. (1996c) 'To the beat of a different drum', *Care Plan*, vol 2, no 4, pp 9-10.

Taylor, R. (1997) 'Funding freedom', Presentation to the Values Into Action Funding Freedom Conference, 19 March.

Taylor, S. (2000) 'An ode to direct payments', *Community Living*, vol 14, no 20, p 7.

Thane, P. (1996) *Foundations of the welfare state* (2nd edn), London: Longman.

Thompson, N., Murphy, M. and Stradling, S. (1994) *Dealing with stress*, Basingstoke: Macmillan.

Thompson, N. (1997) *Anti-discriminatory practice* (2nd edn), Basingstoke: Macmillan.

Thompson, P. (1996) 'Developing direct payments', Paper given at a workshop at the National Social Services Conference, Brighton, 17 October.

Thompson, P. and Lawrence, T. (1996) 'DIG in Parliament', *The DIG Journal*, vol 4, pp 4-7.

Twigg, J. (1998) 'Informal care of older people', in M. Bernard and J. Phillips (eds) *The social policy of old age: Moving into the 21st century*, London: Centre for Policy on Ageing.

Twigg, J. (2000) 'The medical–social boundary and the location of personal care', in A.M. Warnes, L. Warren and M. Nolan (eds) *Care services for late life: Transformations and critique*, London: Jessica Kingsley.

Ungerson, C. (1997) 'Give them the money: is cash a route to empowerment?', *Social Policy and Administration*, vol 31, no 1, pp 45-53.

Unison (2001) *Home care: The forgotten service*, London: Unison.

Valois, N. (1997) 'Direct payments delayed in Ulster', *Community Care*, 3 April, pp 24-30.

Valois, N. (2000a) 'Cash in hand', *Community Care*, 14-20 December, pp 18-19.

Valois, N. (2000b) 'Wanted: caring employees', *Community Care*, 1-7 June, pp 20-1.

Values Into Action (nd) *Decision-making and the law*, London: Values Into Action.

Vasey, S. (2000) *The rough guide to managing personal assistants*, London: NCIL.

Victor, C. (1997) *Community care and older people*, Cheltenham: Stanley Thornes.

Walton, R. (1975) *Women in social work*, London: Routledge and Kegan Paul.

Webb, J. (1996) Kingston's components of success point the way', *Care Plan*, vol 2, no 4, pp 10-11.

Weekers, S. and Pijl, M. (1998) *Home care and care allowances in the European Union*, Utrecht: Netherlands Institute of Care and Welfare.

Wellard, S. (1999) 'The costs of control', *Community Care*, 21-27 January, p 23.

Whitley, P. (1996) 'Growing pains', *Community Care*, 11-17 January, pp 20-1.

Wilson, G. (1994) 'Assembling their own care packages: payments for care by men and women in advanced old age', *Health and Social Care in the Community*, vol 2, pp 283-91.

Witcher, S., Stalker, K., Roadburg, M. and Jones, C. (2000) *Direct payments: The impact on choice and control for disabled people*, Edinburgh: Scottish Executive Central Research Unit.

Zarb, G. (1998) 'What price independence?', Paper presented to the 'Shaping our Futures' Conference, London, 5 June.

Zarb, G. and Nadash, P. (1994) *Cashing in on independence: Comparing the costs and benefits of cash and services*, London: BCODP.

Zarb, G. and Oliver, M. (1993) *Ageing with a disability: What do you expect after all these years?*, London: University of Greenwich.

Zarb, G., Hasler, F., Campbell, J. and Arthur, S. (1997) *Implementation and management of direct payment schemes: First findings – Summary*, London: Policy Studies Institute.

Acts of Parliament/Bills

Care Standards Act 2000

Carers and Disabled Children Act 2000

Community Care (Direct Payments) Act 1996

Disabled Persons (Services) Bill 1992

Disabled Persons (Services) (No 2) Bill 1993

Employment Act 1996

Health and Social Care Act 2001

Health Service and Public Health Act 1968

Mental Health (Patients in the Community) Act 1995

National Assistance Act 1948

National Health Service Act 1977

National Health Service and Community Care Act 1990

Poor Law Amendment Act 1834

Protection of Children Act 1999

Race Relations Act 1976

Sex Discrimination Act 1975

Social Security Act 1986

Social Work (Scotland) Act 1968

Statutory instruments/rules

Statutory Instrument 1996/1923 (NI 19) *The Personal Social Services (Direct Payments) (Northern Ireland) Order 1996*

Statutory Instrument 1997/693 (S 53) *The Community Care (Direct Payments) (Scotland) Regulations 1997*

Statutory Instrument 1997/734 *Community Care (Direct Payments) Regulations 1997*

Statutory Instrument 1997/756 (C 28) *Community Care (Direct Payments) Act 1996 (Commencement) Order 1997*

Statutory Instrument 1997/759 *The Isles of Scilly (Direct Payments Act) Order 1997*

Statutory Instrument 2000/11 *The Community Care (Direct Payments) Amendment Regulations 2000*

Statutory Instrument 2000/1868 (W 127) *The Community Care (Direct Payments) Amendment (Wales) Regulations 2000*

Statutory Instrument 2000/183 *The Community Care (Direct Payments) (Scotland) Amendment Regulations 2000*

Statutory Instrument 2001/441 *The Carers (Services) and Direct Payments (Amendment) (England) Regulations 2001*

Statutory Instrument 2001/442 *The Disabled Children (Direct Payments) (England) Regulations 2001*

Statutory Rule 1997/131 *The Personal Social Services (Direct Payments) Regulations (Northern Ireland) 1997*

Statutory Rule 1997/133 (C 6) *The Personal Social Services (Direct Payments) (1996 Order) (Commencement) Order (Northern Ireland) 1997*

Statutory Rule 2000/114 *The Personal Social Services (Direct Payments) (Amendment) Regulations (Northern Ireland) 2000*

Appendix: Useful resources

All information below is correct at the time of going to press:

Relevant organisations

A range of publications and practical advice leaflets are available from the following organisations:

Advisory, Conciliation and Arbitration Service
For public enquiry points, see www.acas.org.uk/index-6.htm

British Council of Disabled People
Litchurch Plaza
Litchurch Lane
Derby
DE24 8AA

Commission for Racial Equality
Elliot House
10-12 Allington Street
London
SW1E 5EH

The Disablement Income Group
PO Box 5743
Finchingfield
CM7 4PW

Equal Opportunities Commission
Customer Contact Point
Arndale House
Arndale Centre
Manchester
M4 3EQ

The European Network for Independent Living
1 Brennan's Place
Bray
County Wicklow
Ireland

Health and Safety Executive (HSE)
HSE Infoline 08701-545-500

The Independent Living Fund
PO Box 183
Nottingham
NG8 3RD

Inland Revenue
New Employers' Helpline: 0845-60-70-143

The National Centre for Independent Living
250 Kennington Lane
London
SE11 5RD

Values Into Action
Oxford House
Derbyshire Street
London
E2 6HG

Official guidance on direct payments

The Department of Health produces a range of publications and material on direct payments:

- policy and practice guidance (DoH, 1997a, 2000a);
- an accessible introduction for members of the public (DoH, 1998b);
- a multi-media pack for people with learning difficulties (2000b);
- two information videos (DoH, 1998c, 1999);
- speaking notes/overhead templates for presentations on direct payments (DoH, 1997b).

Further guidance is available on the 2000 Carers and Disabled Children Act (DoH, 2001a, b, c, d).

Some of these publications can also be downloaded free of charge from the Department of Health website (see below).

In addition, the Chartered Institute of Public Finance and Accountancy has published financial management guidelines for direct payments (CIPFA, 1998).

Internet resources

The following organisations and websites may contain useful information on direct payments and relevant publications:

BCODP	www.bcodp.org.uk
Community Living	www.community-living.net
Department of Health	www.doh.gov.uk
Disability Archive	www.leeds.ac.uk/disability-studies
European Network on Independent Living	www.independentliving.org/ENIL
Hampshire Direct Payments Scheme	www.hants.gov.uk/socservs/directpayments
Joseph Rowntree Foundation	www.jrf.org.uk
National Centre for Independent Living	www.ncil.org.uk
National Pilot to Promote Independent Living	www.kcl.ac.uk/iahsp
Paradigm	www.paradigm-uk.demon.co.uk
Policy Studies Institute	www.psi.org.uk
Values Into Action	www.viauk.org

Index

I

J

K

L

M

N

O

P

Q

R

S

T

U

V

W

Z

Related reports from The Policy Press

What price independence?
Independent living and people with high support needs

Ann Kestenbaum, The Disablement Income Group

"... easy to read, informative and thought-provoking. It should prove to be a valuable resource for all local authorities and agencies which provide support packages." Therapy Weekly

"... a valuable resource for anyone involved in setting up an independent living scheme ... could also play an important part in stimulating debate as to where the profession sees itself in relation to community care practice in the future." British Journal of Occupational Therapy

PB £13.95 ISBN 1 86134 203 9

Community Care into Practice series

Published in association with the Joseph Rowntree Foundation

Buying independence
Using direct payments to integrate health and social services

Caroline Glendinning, Shirley Halliwell, Sally Jacobs and Kirstein Rummery, National Primary Care Research and Development Centre, University of Manchester, and Jane Tyrer, Health Services Management Unit, University of Manchester

"Social work academics and practice teachers will find this book of value in providing more evidence of user perspectives." Social Work Education

PB £12.99 ISBN 1 86134 225 X

Piloting choice and control for older people
An evaluation

Heather Clark and Jan Spafford, School of Social Studies, University College Chichester

This practical report evaluates an innovative pilot scheme set up to find new ways to deliver services to older people, giving them greater choice and control. Drawing on interviews with older users and care managers involved in the pilot scheme, it looks at older people's perceptions of this scheme and draws out broader lessons for service delivery.

PB £13.95 ISBN 1 86134 243 8

Community Care into Practice series

Published in association with the Joseph Rowntree Foundation

MORE ▶

Also available from The Policy Press

From community care to market care?

The development of welfare services for older people

Robin Means and Hazel Morbey, Faculty of Health and Social Care, University of the West of England, and Randall Smith, School for Policy Studies, University of Bristol

"... a useful addition to the community care literature and should be included on undergraduate reading lists of community care modules." Ian Shaw, Centre for Medical Sociology and Health Policy, University of Nottingham

From community care to market care? focuses on the interpretation and development of national policy at local authority level in four contrasting local authorities. The results of the study will make a significant contribution to our understanding of the community care provision of older people.

PB £18.99 ISBN 1 86134 265 9

HB £45.00 ISBN 1 86134 266 7

From Poor Law to community care

The development of welfare services for elderly people 1939-1971

Robin Means, Faculty of Health and Social Care, University of the West of England and Randall Smith, School for Policy Studies, University of Bristol

Based on extensive research on primary sources and interviews with key actors, this book explores the changing perceptions of the needs of elderly people. It considers the extent to which they have been a priority for resources and looks at the possibilities of policy that combines respect for elderly people with an avoidance of the exploitation of relatives.

PB £18.99 ISBN 1 86134 085 0

HB £45.00 ISBN 1 86134 109 1

For further information about these and other titles published by The Policy Press, please visit our website at: www.policypress.org.uk or telephone +44 (0)117 954 6800

To order, please contact:
Marston Book Services
PO Box 269
Abingdon
Oxon OX14 4YN
UK
Tel: +44 (0)1235 465500
Fax: +44 (0)1235 465556
E-mail: direct-orders@marston.co.uk

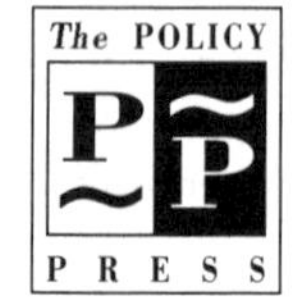